T0296680

CULTURAL ANXIETIES

MEDICAL ANTHROPOLOGY: HEALTH, INEQUALITY, AND SOCIAL JUSTICE

Series editor: Lenore Manderson

Books in the Medical Anthropology series are concerned with social patterns of and social responses to ill health, disease, and suffering, and how social exclusion and social justice shape health and healing outcomes. The series is designed to reflect the diversity of contemporary medical anthropological research and writing, and will offer scholars a forum to publish work that showcases the theoretical sophistication, methodological soundness, and ethnographic richness of the field.

Books in the series may include studies on the organization and movement of peoples, technologies, and treatments; how inequalities pattern access to these; and how individuals, communities and states respond to various assaults on well-being, including from illness, disaster, and violence.

CULTURAL ANXIETIES

Managing Migrant Suffering in France

STÉPHANIE LARCHANCHÉ

RUTGERS UNIVERSITY PRESS

New Brunswick, Camden, and Newark, New Jersey, and London

Library of Congress Cataloging-in-Publication Data
Names: Larchanché, Stéphanie, author.
Title: Cultural anxieties: managing migrant suffering in France /
    Stéphanie Larchanché.
Description: New Brunswick: Rutgers University Press, 2020. | Series: Medical
    anthropology | Includes bibliographical references and index.
Identifiers: LCCN 2019020422 | ISBN 9780813595382 (cloth: alk. paper) |
    ISBN 9780813595375 (paperback: alk. paper)
Subjects: | MESH: Centre Françoise Minkowska (Paris, France) | Mental Health
    Services | Ethnopsychology—methods | Emigrants and Immigrants—psychology |
    Culturally Competent Care | Stress, Psychological | France
Classification: LCC RC450.F7 | NLM WA 305 GF7 | DDC 362.2/10944361—dc23
LC record available at https://lccn.loc.gov/2019020422

A British Cataloging-in-Publication record for this book is available from the
British Library.

♾ The paper used in this publication meets the requirements of the American
National Standard for Information Sciences—Permanence of Paper for Printed
Library Materials, ANSI Z39.48-1992.

www.rutgersuniversitypress.org

Manufactured in the United States of America

For my daughter, Julia
And for my husband, Zanga

CONTENTS

FOREWORD

LENORE MANDERSON

Medical Anthropology: Health, Inequality and Social Justice is a new series from Rutgers University Press, designed to capture the diversity of contemporary medical anthropological research and writing. The beauty of ethnography is its capacity, through storytelling, to make sense of suffering as a social experience, and to set it in context. This series is concerned with health and illness, and inequality and social justice, and central to this are the ways that social structures and ideologies shape the likelihood and impact of infections, injuries, bodily ruptures and disease, chronic conditions and disability, treatment and care, and social repair and death.

The brief for this series is broad. The books are concerned with health and illness, healing practices, and access to care, but the authors illustrate, too, the importance of context—of geography, physical condition, service availability, and income. Health and illness are social facts; the circumstances of the maintenance and loss of health are always and everywhere shaped by structural, global, and local relations. Society, culture, economy, and political organization as much as ecology shape the variance of illness, disability, and disadvantage. But as medical anthropologists have long illustrated, the relationships between social context and health status are complex. In addressing these questions, the authors in this series showcase the theoretical sophistication, methodological rigor, and empirical richness of the field, while expanding a map of illness and social and institutional life to illustrate the effects of material conditions and social meanings in troubling and surprising ways.

The books in the series move across social circumstances, health conditions, and geography, as well as their intersections and interactions, to demonstrate how individuals, communities, and states manage assaults on well-being. The books reflect medical anthropology as a constantly changing field of scholarship, drawing diversely on research in residential and virtual communities, clinics, and laboratories; in emergency care and public health settings; among service providers, individual healers, and households; and within social bodies, human bodies, and biology. While medical anthropology once concentrated on systems of healing, particular diseases, and embodied experiences, today the field has expanded to include environmental disaster and war; science, technology, and faith; gender-based violence; and forced migration. Curiosity about the body and its vicissitudes remains a pivot for our work, but our concerns are with the location of bodies in social life, and with how social structures, temporal imperatives, and shifting exigencies shape life courses. This dynamic field reflects an ethics of the discipline to address these pressing issues of our time.

Globalization has contributed to and adds to the complexity of influences on health outcomes; it (re)produces social and economic relations that institutionalize poverty, unequal conditions of everyday life and work, and environments in which diseases increase or subside. Globalization patterns the movement and relations of peoples, technologies and knowledge, and programs and treatments; it shapes differences in health experiences and outcomes across space; and it informs and amplifies inequalities at individual and country levels. Global forces and local inequalities compound and constantly load on individuals to affect their physical and mental health, as well as their households and communities. At the same time, as the subtitle of this series indicates, we are concerned with questions of social exclusion and inclusion, social justice, and repair—again both globally and in local settings. The books will challenge readers to reflect not only on sickness and suffering, deficits, and despair, but also on resistance and restitution—on how people respond to injustices and evade the fault lines that might seem to predetermine life outcomes. While not all of the books take this direction, the aim is to widen the frame within which we conceptualize embodiment and suffering.

Over one in ten people in France are born outside the country, and with their children, around one-fifth of all people come from immigrant backgrounds, including various former French colonies. The vast majority of immigrants are now from North African, sub-Saharan, and Turkish and Middle Eastern backgrounds, and live in Paris, the tentative end of journeys precipitated by environmental decay, economic decline, violence, and poverty, and by aspirations for different pathways for their descendants, if not for themselves. The routes by which they travel to France are varied—a mix of formal immigration, visa extensions and overstays, and country entry by stealth. Across the city and countrywide, various hospitals and clinics seek to provide mental as well as physical care for people from these diverse populations.

Mode of entry to France, the legitimacy (or not) of continued residence, and economic precarity are not why immigrants end up with mental health problems and in need of acute and ongoing care; likewise, social and cultural backgrounds—differences in faith, tradition, and language—are not reasons for care. People's care needs mirror those of French citizens, even if in the context of mental health in particular, experiences of extreme suffering in their countries of birth and during and after migration have a particularly strong impact. However, economic and educational disparities, differences in faith and interpretations of distress, and difficulties in communication and comprehension in clinical and other settings all interfere with access to and the uptake and effectiveness of clinical care and advice for people whose lives are made liminal because of their undocumented migrant status and rejection as asylum seekers. People without papers are stuck in a borderland that makes everyday living and sense-making deeply troubling.

Stéphanie Larchanché is the director of Research, Teaching and Professional Training at Centre Minkowska and was originally employed to provide training in "cultural competence" and to review, support, and evaluate clinical encounters. The Centre Minkowska, the setting of this ethnography, is a transcultural psychiatry clinic in Paris, established by psychiatrist Eugène Minkowski with the aim to improve health-care access by and services provided to immigrants. In *Cultural Anxieties*, Stéphanie Larchanché explores through the analytic of anxiety the logic behind the center's establishment and operation, and the reasoning behind migrant patients' referrals to the center. Center staff must negotiate the provision of culturally sensitive care to patients with French republican ideals of universality. The flow between cultural difference and mental illness and distress leads to a notion of "migrant suffering," creating the need for clinics like Centre Minkowska to provide specialized care.

Stéphanie Larchanché draws on both her doctoral research at the center and her later employment at the center—including her most recent work as a psychotherapist in training—to describe and analyze patients' experiences of everyday life, which constitutes the background that they bring, as clients, to the center. Larchanché writes from "the borderland"—as an anthropologist outsider and psychotherapist insider. She writes of the borderland, too—of the center as a public health institution and as an NGO operating independently of the state system. The center's clients are also border dwellers, forced to work around, and often with, the administrative tangles of asylum status; residency; and the rights to work, housing, education, and health care. Caught in the nowhere of state bureaucracy, people are socially marginalized, causing distress for some and compounding preexisting suffering for others. Health-care providers, including in this context psychologists, counselors, social workers, and psychotherapists, work to help clients learn to live with the uncertainties of this borderland life. But as Larchanché illustrates, this is especially difficult when the supportive scaffolding of the state and the NGO is also uncertain, leaving service organizations and agencies to struggle with staff shortages, limited training, and budgetary constraints, which limits access to interpreters to negotiate care and support. Both health-care providers and their clients, and others working to link up services, struggle in this borderland on a daily basis. In this beautifully compelling account of an institution, its staff, and its clients, we engage with the challenges of social suffering, state responsibility, institutional engagement, and contemporary ethics.

ABBREVIATIONS

AMC	Clinical Medical Anthropology
AME	State Medical Aid (for the undocumented who have been residing in France for over three months)
ASE	Child Protection Services
CADA	Center for Asylum Seekers
CAO	(Temporary) Housing and Orientation Center
CASO	Health Care and Orientation Center (managed by Médecins du monde)
CLIS	School Inclusion Class
CMP	Mental Health Center
CMU	Universal Healthcare Coverage (accessible to asylum seekers during their application process)
CNDA	National Court for Asylum Seekers
DNA	National Housing System
EPP	Evaluation of Professional Practices
EMPP	Mobile Psychiatry Teams for Situations of Extreme Precarity
HAS	French National Health Authority
ISM	Inter-Migrant Services
MDPH	Departmental Houses for Disabled Persons
OFII	French Office for Immigration and Integration
OFPRA	Office for the Protection of Refugees and Stateless Persons
PASS	Healthcare Access Platform (for poor, uninsured, or undocumented patients)
PMI	Center for Mother and Infant Protection
RASED	Special Aid Network for Students with Difficulties
SSAE	Social Service for Support to Emigrants
TEF	Therapist in Training
UPE2A	Pedagogical Unit for Arriving Non-francophone Pupils
ZEP/REP	Priority Education Zone/Priority Education Network
ZUP	Priority Urban Zone

CULTURAL ANXIETIES

INTRODUCTION

Paris, Winter 2015. Terrorist attacks on the headquarters of the French satirical newspaper *Charlie Hebdo* have just occurred. The country is shaken, and people across France mourn the journalists who have died. They are upheld as icons of republican freedom and secular values, and the political response is rapid: the current prime minister, Manuel Valls, unveils a plan to fight terrorism and radical Islam at home and abroad, including increased surveillance. Meanwhile, media headlines regularly proclaim that an "immigration crisis" is hitting Europe, which fuels existing fears linked to economic insecurity and global terrorism.

In this context, Moussa, aged sixteen and from Mali, arrived in France illegally and was referred to Centre Minkowska. Centre Minkowska is a transcultural psychiatry clinic, catering specifically to migrants and located in the seventeenth arrondissement of Paris. It is where I have been working as an applied anthropologist since 2010. The referral letter was sent by a psychologist at the children's social housing institution where Moussa resided, in an outer suburb of Paris. It mentioned Moussa's "depressive state and integration difficulties." The psychologist and the institution's educational team were concerned about his psychological fragility and permanent state of sadness: "He never smiles." During one interview, the psychologist claimed that he seemed "annoyed" by her questions about the reasons he had come to France. She noted that his father had died in 2011, and Moussa left his home following a dispute with his paternal uncles about his father's heritage. He expressed that his priorities were to access professional training, get a job as quickly as possible, and send money to his family back home. She commented that this "mission he imposed on himself" caused him to refuse any form of enjoyment.

The psychologist's letter mentioned that Moussa was in a class for non-French speakers and seemed eager to learn. However, the psychologist continued:

> Even though he showed an interest to integrate the group further, what we are observing is that he has not established any close relationship with either his peers or adults. He often appears irritable, tending to isolate himself in his bedroom to get away from the group. On a daily basis, we observed difficulties, or even a reluctance

to adapt to cultural practices that are different from his. Moussa now refuses to shake hands with women to greet them. In terms of diet, as he only accepts halal food, he simply refuses to consume meat, and during a recent meal, he refused to use silverware and ate with his fingers. This makes Moussa suffer, as he is left with feelings of misunderstanding and even anger towards the educators who regularly try to discuss these issues with him.

Given these observations and Moussa's apparent reluctance to "the idea of opening up to a person culturally different from him," the psychologist recommended psychological support with an ethnopsychiatric approach as "appropriate."

Upon reading the referral letter, impressions among MEDIACOR participants—the referral unit at Centre Minkowska—were mixed. (MEDIACOR is an acronym standing for *MEDIation, ACcueil, ORientation*. The organization and logics of MEDIACOR meetings will be detailed in chapter 2.) Some anticipated that the referral would stigmatize Moussa, whose behavior was likely the object of the housing staff's anxieties and projected negative representations rather than an actual clinical concern. Others, including Minkowska's leading psychiatrist, argued that there was no way to ascertain whether that was the case—even though the framing of the referring psychologist's arguments raised red flags—and that our responsibility was to determine whether Moussa needed our help. He also noted that Moussa, as a recent arrival in France, was unlikely to be seen by a psychiatrist in a "mainstream" district mental health institution. In the end, an evaluation session was scheduled at the Centre. However, Moussa did not show at this first appointment.

The staff at his housing institution gave no reason for Moussa's absence, but an educator called the Centre back to reschedule his appointment. On the second try, Moussa arrived in the company of a young educator who was new to his case. As Moussa entered the room, he readily shook our hands—three of us were women, the psychiatrist a man. Moussa said he did not know why he had been sent to the Centre but that he had been compelled by the housing institution's staff. The Centre's psychiatrist explained the psychologist's referral letter, and Moussa was astonished, noting that he had met with her only once. He asked us why she had referred him, and we discussed her concern that he was withdrawn at the residence. He told us that was simply his way of being (*c'est ma façon d'être*), that he was like that at home, and that he did not need help for it. We then asked questions about why he came to France and about his daily life here. He explained that he was from a village in the Kayes region of Mali, had attended "Arabic school," and continued to practice Arabic in private by reading novels or the Quran; he did not want to forget that language.[1] However, he noted that he also reads the *Bescherelle*, a standard French grammar textbook, to practice French and studies in a French as a Foreign Language (FLE) class, which he finds challenging: the students are all at different levels, and some speak no French. At his residence, he shares a room with a young Pakistani boy who speaks only English, and they communicate using gestures. He revealed that it is important for him to maintain fluency in Arabic because this symbolically ties him to his late father. He told us about poems he wrote in Arabic and then tried to translate into French; the last one he wrote was about a day trip on the Champs-Elysées. Moussa told us that no one at his residence was aware of his writings except for a woman named Aminata, with whom he shared some poems and who once offered him a book in Arabic.

Nothing disturbing emerged from our interview with Moussa. He did not wish to see a psychologist at the moment. Rather, he wanted professional training to become a mail carrier or to work as a security officer, and he reported that he had researched existing job possibilities. At the end of our evaluation interview and with Moussa's agreement, we asked the educator who had accompanied him to rejoin us. When we asked whether she wanted to relay more of her colleagues' concerns about Moussa, she timidly confessed that she hardly knew him. She had only recently started working at the residence and was unaware of the others' concerns. In fact, her impression of Moussa was positive. We ended by telling Moussa he could contact the Centre if he ever felt the need to speak with a mental health professional. After he and his educator left, we spent a few minutes sharing our impressions.

Discrepancies like this are common at Minkowska, and MEDIACOR evaluation sessions were created specifically to address them. That day, we all agreed it was the intersection of the residence staff's subjective representations around Moussa's culture, his religious convictions, and his personality that combined to create the psychologist's portrait of him as experiencing psychological distress. The MEDIACOR team easily identified the influence of social representations from the colonial imaginary, current anxieties around youth radicalization, and clichés about unaccompanied minors on the residence staff's interpretation of Moussa's behavior. To the list of things that contributed to Moussa's mischaracterization by the residence staff, I would add structural determinants, such as host institutions' lack of resources to provide quality support, the growing number of children within such residences, a high staff-turnover rate, and a critical lack of training to help staff members deal with the complexities around unaccompanied minors. The Minkowska team concluded that in contrast to the residence staff's assessment, Moussa was experiencing a quite positive acculturation process and employing creative adaptive strategies to maintain relationships with his family and culture of origin, such as writing poetry in Arabic. Moussa was actively cultivating a healthy integration strategy, despite what the professionals who worked with him at the residence seemed to think.

For those of us at Centre Minkowska, it appeared that a combination of the residence staff's negative social representations, a historically situated context of migrant-related anxiety in France, Moussa's personal difficulties in relating with others, and a host of structural issues all contributed to the pathologizing of Moussa's behavior. This raises important questions: How could an evaluation interview with Centre Minkowska's professionals yield such clearly different results from one by the psychologist at Moussa's residence? Why did Moussa's education team send an educator to the appointment who barely knew him and was unable to provide any background information or context for his situation? Equally important, what is the broader social role of transcultural clinicians at Centre Minkowska, who are identified by other institutions as experts in charge of migrants' suffering? How do these professionals deal with such stigmatizing referrals in their daily practice? How do they define and legitimize their expertise? What are the responsibilities of transcultural clinicians to confront and change the unjust systems of power in which they are embedded?

This is an ethnography about Centre Minkowska, a transcultural psychiatry clinic where I have been working as an applied anthropologist since 2010. In this ethnography, then, I am both an observer and a participant. I write from a position at "the borderland": as a staff member, I am involved in clinical activities, but as an anthropologist, I maintain a commitment to decentered observation of my colleagues, my institution, and my own positionality. This book offers a unique take on how cultural competence is construed and applied at Centre Minkowska, under a republican model that finds it difficult to acknowledge cultural diversity. I consider how the clinical medical anthropology approach and its focus on person-centered care in transcultural psychiatry are deeply intertwined with the Centre's historical foundations, the personalities of the people who work there, and the constraints imposed by the local public health system. I rely on MEDIACOR meetings—the triage unit for the referral of patients at Centre Minkowska—as a privileged vantage point from which to observe and analyze the enactment of cultural competence. My goal is to analyze how the anxieties experienced by staff at the Centre reflect broader anxieties of contemporary French society and of global society as well. Therefore, my reference to cultural anxieties is polysemic.

First, it refers to anxieties experienced by staff at specialized mental health clinics. By "specialized," I refer in my own terms to culturally sensitive clinics catering specifically to immigrant populations. I use this term as an analytic to pragmatically group mental health institutions that cater to migrants regardless of their clinical approach (e.g., ethnopsychiatry, transcultural psychiatry, or intercultural psychology). I describe how specialized mental health experts negotiate tensions between French republican ideals of universality, which downplay differences of race or ethnicity, and their desire to provide culturally sensitive care to their patients. This encompasses the anxieties such agents experience as they work at the edges of the system and seek to fill gaps created by dysfunctional social infrastructures. They intervene in what is known in social theory as "zones of abandonment" (Biehl 2005). This is particularly true for clinicians working with undocumented migrants and rejected asylum seekers. I use the polysemic notion of "cultural anxieties" to specifically explore logics behind migrant patients' referrals to a transcultural psychiatry clinic in Paris, Centre Minkowska. In the research for this book, I discovered that state agents in the mental health field often characterize migrants' difficult experiences with integration—or simple expressions of cultural difference—as a particular kind of "suffering" that was not the purview of mainstream mental health but rather the responsibility of institutions like Centre Minkowska. Here I thus focus on how social anxieties may lead state agents to interpret expressions of cultural difference as socially deviant—or as examples of mental suffering or pathology. I suggest that state agents use social representations and discourse to draw parallels between cultural difference and pathology. In doing so, they build legitimate ground on which to validate their ideas about how "migrant suffering" requires care from "expert" clinics like Centre Minkowska.

Second, "cultural anxieties" refers to anxieties that contemporary state agents—across institutional realms—experience when faced with limited means to provide support to newly arrived migrants in the process of "regularization" and to older residents who continue to face social and economic challenges. With this use of the term, I touch on the limits of the French welfare state and its increasing disengagement from immigration issues since the 1970s and the end of *les trente glorieuses*, or the thirty glorious years of postwar economic prosperity. Anxieties in this context are about endless administrative delays in processing visas or asylum status, which leave people in states of social liminality; chronic staff shortages, such as those within asylum seekers' housing centers, which have only one psychologist who visits on one day per week; and budgetary constraints that prevent funding, training, and creating policies for professional language interpreters to work in public services. These anxieties concern both statutory refugees who remain homeless and freshly arrived migrant youth, who often experience traumatic immigration trajectories marked by confusion and constraint. They may not speak French or may find themselves grouped together in an "integration" class with a teacher who lacks the resources to teach them. This systemic lack of support produces suffering. Without the means to address such structural suffering, state agents—the psychologist working at the asylum seekers' housing center, the social worker struggling to find emergency housing for a family whose asylum application was rejected—may find it useful to reframe structural suffering as "cultural suffering" or to rely on "experts on migrants" in their search for support for their clients.

Ultimately, the anxieties of both clinicians and state agents relate to the broad anxieties French social actors experience in the face of sociodemographic change and economic insecurity. These anxieties have deep roots in stigmatizing representations of cultural difference, formed during France's colonial past and inherited from scientific discourse produced in the context of both colonial psychiatry and French ethnopsychiatry in the 1970s (for more, see Fassin 2000). Such representations remain common within the French social imaginary, and anxieties have only intensified over the past three decades with increased migration and consequent changes in the French demographic landscape. More recently, certain events have increased these anxieties: suburban riots in 2005 and 2007, when second-generation North and sub-Saharan African youth expressed discontent toward French institutional resistance to their integration; the influx of fleeing Syrians since 2012, which has led to a media-deemed "refugee crisis"; and terrorist attacks perpetrated by second-generation French Muslims. The French government interpreted these successive events as threats to France's national identity, and populist parties have capitalized on that. In recent contexts, the latter depicted migrants and their children as the ultimate threat to the nation's integrity.

Beyond the French context, anxiety permeates many people's experience of the contemporary world: growing social and economic inequalities favor the rise of populist and nationalist movements in wealthier nations; natural catastrophes and armed conflicts result in millions of displaced people; and global terrorism is invoked daily in news media. In such times of fear and uncertainty, identity politics tend to emerge: Who are we? Where are we heading? Who will protect us? Lines between those who belong and those who do not often harden. While this dynamic is universal, people in each nation or group draw those lines differently and reflect their own histories and ideologies in the process. Race, ethnicity, and religion are common markers of difference, and social representations that have evolved around them—while shaped by historical context—often travel across time. Anxieties that stem from fear in the face of social change or difference are culturally shaped, and almost without us realizing it, they recurrently crystallize around people who are considered "other"—migrants and their children.

Anxieties are both social and subjective. Specialized mental health centers like Centre Minkowska have become the theater where these anxieties converge and are enacted. While they are part of the system, such centers function at the margins and provide a space where alternative interpretations of suffering are possible and where people's humanity is acknowledged. As such, they constitute a unique vantage from which to observe social struggles that have economic and political roots; their presence relates to the failure and unwillingness of the state to deal with processes of change that began with the industrial revolution, colonial imperialism, and the onset of labor migration and continue in the present. The centers also provide opportunities to raise questions as to the contradictions and limits of their existence within the national public health system—particularly the constant tension between their mission of care and the regulating system in which they are inevitably caught and in which they indirectly participate. This tension produces a set of anxieties, negotiated daily by specialized mental health professionals, that rest at the heart of this book.

THE RESEARCH

This book is the fruit of two branches of research. The first is my dissertation field-work, conducted over eighteen months between 2007 and 2008, in which I compared mental health-care discourse and practice within three specialized clinics in Paris. The second relies on the accumulated knowledge and experience I have acquired during these past years as I practiced anthropology at Centre Minkowska.

During my dissertation fieldwork in Paris from March 2007 to June 2008, the country's political context was particularly sensitive. I arrived on the eve of Nicolas Sarkozy's election to the presidency in April 2007. His victory was due largely to a campaign focused heavily on national security and identity. This 2007 presidential campaign capitalized on fears felt by many in the aftermath of the 2005 Paris suburban riots and the resulting negative, stigmatizing representations produced around visible French minorities—youth of North and sub-Saharan African origin—and immigration in general (Tshimanga, Gondola, and Bloom 2009). In the context of extremely restrictive immigration policies, I witnessed a fact already analyzed elsewhere (Fassin 2001; Ticktin 2011): the right to health care could constitute a last resort for residence legitimacy. I was also ideally positioned to document how the interactions of intangible factors—social stigmatization, precarious living conditions, and the climate of fear and suspicion generated by anti-immigration policies—hindered undocumented migrants' access to health care. These factors produced powerful subjectivation effects in that they not only negatively influenced social representations of migrants as undeserving of care—thereby affecting some health professionals' ethics—but also negatively influenced migrants' understanding of themselves as deserving of access to care (Larchanché 2012).

After I felt sufficiently immersed in the field context, I selected three mental health institutions that I considered representative of the main theoretical approaches to specialized mental health in France at the time. Among these, Centre Minkowska, a transcultural psychiatry clinic, had developed a clinical medical anthropology approach to the provision of mental health care. The Centre exemplifies what is called a "second-intention" clinic in French public health jargon: it receives "foreign patients" who fall through gaps produced when a broad array of state agents (from the education, justice, and public health sectors) consider patients' problems cultural and therefore outside their professional competence or ability to help. During my early observations, I noted that referrals to specialized mental health clinics could be arbitrary or even occur before any other institutional measures were attempted. This made me question how such specialized centers are used in practice; they seemed to be designated by many state agents as places to deal with cultural difference in ways that "mainstream" institutions could not. Referral narratives, as well as meetings between referring state agents and clinical staff—more than mental health care delivery to migrant patients per se—became my central interest.

This prompted me to collect data along unexpected research directions. In particular, I was taken to places outside the clinic. Conversations about and around the clinic became as relevant as clinical interactions. Research on this path entailed tracking diffuse relations not only within medical institutions but among a wide array of state-sponsored ones. It also involved mastering multiple institutional languages and a battery of acronyms. The most challenging aspect of my fieldwork was tracing referrals; I was able to witness only a small portion of the referring processes for patients at my three field sites. To better understand and frame health-care providers' rationales for referrals, I had to devise a method to trace the circulation of participants' voices and delineate relevant institutional networks. I ended up tracking three major domains: the referral's origin (school, legal services, social services); the official rationale for referrals, which was located in patients' files; and pre-consultation meetings. At Minkowska, where I had access to patients' files, I compiled information on referrals' origins and official rationales within a table.[2] As often as possible, I attended pre-consultation meetings, which were not a systematic feature of the management of Minkowska's patients. Such meetings primarily occurred when referring actors were still debating whether or not to refer their "patient" to the center. These exchanges were particularly illuminating because they offered the most direct and unmediated discourse on the relevance of cultural difference in the expression of mental health pathologies or on the correlation actors may draw between cultural difference and the ambiguous notion of "difficulty"—a concept used relentlessly in conversations about what was characterized as immigrant patients' "problems."

Early on, I realized how anxiety-ridden the field of specialized mental health could be for professionals, not just patients. First, clinicians actively defined their practice and theoretical approach in contrast to ethnopsychiatry. As the study of disorders in their cultural context, ethnopsychiatry emerged in the climate of colonialism and problematically relied on the racial and cultural stereotypes disseminated during that period through the practice of colonial psychiatry in particular (Fassin and Rechtman 2005). While ethnopsychiatry evolved to integrate more critical approaches that aimed at deconstructing essentializing understandings of cultural difference, it remains debated because of its colonial roots (Beneduce 2006). At the close of the 1970s in France, psychologist Tobie Nathan proposed a new approach to ethnopsychiatry, which targeted migrants specifically. This approach emphasized cultural otherness and "traditional" etiologies (Nathan 1994) at the expense of both psychiatric knowledge and consideration for the social determinants of mental health (Fassin 2000b). Public debates about this culturalist approach negatively affected perceptions of the field of specialized mental health, especially in a republican state, where the term "culturalist" may be considered an ultimate insult. At Centre Minkowska, professionals were not the direct heirs of Tobie Nathan's ethnopsychiatry approach, but like others, they had been swayed during the heyday of ethnopsychiatry, which inevitably affected their clinical practice. In countless conversations, specialized mental health professionals justified to me how their approach was distinctive. Although over a decade had passed since the demise of the Ethnopsychiatry School (Fassin and Rechtman 2005), feelings of uneasiness were still vivid among the professionals with whom I worked.

Referral narratives at Centre Minkowska were also an expression of many state agents' anxieties about cultural difference—how to name it, deal with it, and manage migrants and their children. Whether I met state agents at the clinic for preconsultation visits, interacted within their own institutional walls, or read their referral letters, I noticed how their justifications of differential treatment—referring an individual to a "specialized" institution rather than a mainstream mental health center—relied on complex, culturally coherent discursive strategies to legitimize their rationales. These professionals' referrals to specialized institutions were often the result of their ambivalence about how to handle certain situations. For example, there were situations in which the representations of suffering expressed by patients challenged professionals' ability to respond appropriately; I witnessed this when a mother left her children with child services because she felt they were possessed by evil spirits who threatened her life on a daily basis. At other times, I observed that state agents who refer people to Centre Minkowska did so when faced with the limits of their own institutions and professional missions. For instance, a social worker who accompanied an asylum seeker whose request was rejected, and for whom institutional support was no longer available, might turn to specialized mental health as a last resort—even if the individual did not express a need to engage in psychotherapy. In fact, I found that a significant proportion of individuals referred to specialized mental health centers had not been consulted about their referral, as Moussa's situation illustrated. Professionals' representations of cultural difference and structural determinants are often conflated in patients' referrals, and difference is used as an alibi to legitimize the referral. In Moussa's case, the internal lack of communication between this young man and the housing residence staff directly derives from the shortage of psychologists in such institutions and their inability to cope with clients' demand or needs, together with the high turnover rate for educators working in child protection services: Moussa had only met the psychologist once, shortly upon his arrival at the residence, and the educator who accompanied him to Minkowska barely knew him, as she had just started the job. The housing residence staff's lack of acquaintance with Moussa likely prevented them from sketching a more complex and nuanced portrait of him and from alleviating their anxieties about the danger he represented to them.

The result is that a wide variety of migrants' situations are being handled by specialized mental health professionals, even though not all of them actually require mental health care or culturally sensitive expertise. In turn—as MEDIACOR staff's ambivalent response to Moussa's referral letter illustrates—this leads to internal debates about which referrals should be relevant to Centre Minkowska's expertise and whose responsibility it is to care for migrants, and under which circumstances. Is cultural difference a legitimate reason to refer a patient? If yes, is accepting a referral on the basis of cultural difference stigmatizing for the patient? If no, what situations *are* legitimate for referral? Is a language barrier between patients and stage agents enough to motivate a referral? If not, in which situations would it be so? What exactly is it that "mainstream" mental health institutions lack that the Centre is able to provide?

WORKING FROM THE BORDERLAND

In 2010, after completing my doctoral research, I was offered a part-time position at Centre Minkowska as the coordinator of the Research and Teaching Department.[3] I am now full-time director of this department. It is unusual for a relatively small medical institution like Centre Minkowska, unaffiliated with a university, to be engaged in research and teaching activities or to hire an anthropologist. Indeed, my professional qualification is classified as "psychologist" on the payroll system. Hiring me was a strategic move: my presence as a *medical* anthropologist (the staff often insisted I introduce myself thus) validated the clinical medical anthropology approach that was advocated by members of the Centre and adopted in 1999, partly to distinguish the Centre from others in the field. The founder of this approach in France, psychiatrist and anthropologist Rachid Bennegadi, dedicated his career to improving health-care access for migrants in France. My appointment was also the result of a directorship that believes in the importance of reflexivity regarding one's activities and reframing them within a social and structural context in a bid to improve health-care access and delivery. For several years, my job partly involved coordinating and teaching a one-year continuing education program, which was created in 2007 in partnership with Université Paris Descartes to train students and general business professionals in an approach to service provision called "cultural competence." The rest of the time, I attended patient evaluation sessions and staff meetings, called MEDIACOR meetings, and took notes on their proceedings. Regular meetings—those which did not involve patient evaluations—were audio-recorded. My analysis in this book is based on such notes, audio data, and participant observation.

In 2014, I committed to furthering my understanding of mental health disorders and treatment and enrolled in a psychotherapy program. About a year later, Rachid Bennegadi suggested I start seeing patients as a psychotherapist-in-training and under his supervision. While my doctoral fieldwork primarily focused on representations of immigrants through patient referrals, my years employed at the Centre have brought me closer to their everyday experiences in enriching and humbling ways. I am regularly in awe of patients' strength and resilience, and working full time at the clinic and practicing psychotherapy have challenged theoretical frames I learned as a social scientist. My professional work has nuanced my understanding of those frames, and my goal in this book is to capture and explore this kind of real-world complexity. Over these last few years, I descended from the metaphorical ivory tower and engaged with the practical messiness of institutional life. Today, as an anthropologist and a psychotherapist, a participant-observer and staff member, I write from a position at the borderland. In fact, I suggest that Centre Minkowska itself constitutes a borderland: as a public health institution, it is inside the system, but it also falls outside, through its status and management as an association.

Because I am a Centre staff member, you may question my capacity to produce data deemed objective or to maintain a professional level of distance within my research. I have always questioned the positivist approach to science and its claims to objectivity. With this ethnography, I attempt to define the contours of a critical praxis (Wilkinson and Kleinman 2016) based not on distance but on reflexivity. Across the pages that follow, I share my ethical anxieties around the ambiguities of my work and my proximity to research participants, and I unambiguously resort to the pronoun *we*. This is intentional; I have known some colleagues at Minkowska for almost a decade, and some have become friends. But I see no ambiguity in my position as both a colleague and a critical observer. Staff at Minkowska have always known about this book project and embraced it with full consent. Any anxiety about it was more mine than theirs.

OUTLINE OF THE BOOK

This book is divided into three parts, which I delineate here from a theoretical standpoint. The first part, "The Context," includes two chapters and addresses the social frame within which the notion of migrant suffering is deployed in mental health care in France. The second part, "Referral Narratives and Ethical Double-Binds," includes two chapters and analyzes referral narratives and the ethical deliberations that take place at Centre Minkowska. The last part, "Ethical Deliberations," includes three chapters and reflects on the praxis that emerges from Centre Minkowska's cultural competence framework.

In chapter 1, "A Genealogy of 'Migrant Suffering,'" I draw on the Foucauldian concept of genealogy (1970) to analyze the production of social discourse around the notion of migrant suffering. I define *migrant suffering* as the socially constructed discursive product of a mental health care field that caters specifically to migrants. However, this does not imply that the concept refers to something unreal; experiences of exile, stigmatization, and social precarity to which many migrants are vulnerable certainly engender psychological suffering and produce ill health. My goal is to understand when and why the notion of migrant suffering gained social legitimacy and became the object of specialized mental health initiatives sponsored by the state.

I use the category "migrants" to employ a perspective-neutral terminology that avoids other political categories often used to sanction people's motives to migrate in terms of social and political legitimacy—such as "labor migrant," "sans-papiers" (undocumented migrant), or "refugee." I use the "suffering" category equally intentionally; it is in tune with the politicized language of *social suffering* born in the 1980s, and it refers to the vague ways in which state agents have come to define psychic suffering—without necessarily resorting to clinical or medical nosology (Jacques 2004). This is important to note, since this vagueness of language potentially masks the social inequalities and the forms of exclusion that lie at the very root of this suffering.

Part of my analysis is temporal. I address the evolution of scientific discourse in the management of racial and cultural difference in mental health initiatives in the French colonies and in France. By approaching the bodies of migrants as political—as sites of power and control (Comaroff 1985, 1993; Hunt 1999; Lock and Scheper-Hughes 1996)—I unveil the dialectical interaction between political strategies of control and the creation of scientific categories that stigmatize the "other" in morally sanctioned ways. In the past, sociologists and anthropologists (Bourdieu 1996; Durkheim 1973; Durkheim and Mauss 1963) have shown how such disciplines of the body guarantee social relations of dominance, sustain sovereign forms of power, and become normative social structures that are embodied in mental structures over time. The arbitrariness of such knowledge is thus forgotten, which creates a habitus of social perception—or knowledge that "goes without saying"—around the meanings behind racial and cultural difference (Bourdieu 1977) and the powerful symbolic systems that articulate such difference through everyday language (Bourdieu 1991). In this book, I examine how migrant subjectivities are socially constructed; travel through time; and are reproduced, contested, or negotiated through the scientific discourse of specialized mental health.

In contemporary France, the psychological suffering of migrants has received increasing scholarly and media attention since the late 1970s, which corresponds to the end of labor migration and the tightening of controls around economic migration and asylum policies. The development of a specialized field of mental health expertise paralleled this interest and reflects broader shifts in the contemporary moral economy (Fassin and Rechtman 2009). This concept of "moral economy" refers to the "study of the production, circulation and appropriation of norms and values, sensibilities and emotions" (Fassin 2012, 13) in a given context and at a given time. Recently, the notion of suffering has been understood as the product of sociopolitical conditions, which are defined as "structural violence" (Farmer 1996) or "the violence of everyday life" (Scheper-Hughes 1993). This theoretical shift has come to constitute a new ethical regime within scholarship (Das et al. 2000; Das 2001; Kleinman, Das, and Lock 1997).

My work engages with recent theorizations on "the suffering body" in the context of French immigration policies (Sayad 1999, 2004; Fassin 2005; Ticktin 2011). Didier Fassin (2005) was the first to elaborate on the tension between moral economies of repression and compassion in relation to changing social representations around migrants. He showed how nation-states shifted their policies at the end of the Cold War toward heavily controlling migration in the wake of "a new world order" (Fassin 2005, 373) characterized by exacerbated nationalisms and increased population movement. French officials, until then relatively sympathetic to asylum seekers, began questioning the motives and the legitimacy of all incoming migrants. The government began characterizing all categories of migrants through negative social representations, such as *clandestins* (illegal) and illegitimate. The only exception was within the domain of health, in which broader moral values of care and compassion helped sustain the legitimacy of migrants as "apolitical" suffering bodies (Ticktin 2011). However, as anthropologist Miriam Ticktin skillfully demonstrates, this moral legitimation of the suffering body led to new political forms of regulation and to the reproduction of existing forms of gendered, racialized inequalities rather than affirming a new logic of care.

Cultural Anxieties explores how these processes of biolegitimacy play out in the context of mental health in France. In this ethnography, I focus on the institutional discourse of specialized mental health care and on how staff members in these institutions manage the stigmatizing referrals they receive. Alternatively, I pay attention to how referring state agents name, interpret, and handle cultural difference through social services and the identification of "migrant suffering."

Following this frame of analysis, in chapter 2, "Transcultural Practice at Centre Minkowska," I describe how Centre Minkowska developed and gained legitimacy within the field of specialized mental health care, and the tensions it met in the process. I focus on how France's ideological context and the recent managerial policies in health care underpinned Centre Minkowska's choice of a clinical medical anthropology approach to mental health care as a way to destigmatize the patient-clinician encounter and to better evaluate clinical practice through public health standards. This approach takes culture into account in therapy, and it strives to achieve a middle-ground position between defining all pathologies as culturally determined, which leads to patients' stigmatization, and providing culture-blind care, which leads to ethnocentrism. It highlights the cultural nature of the clinical encounter between two explanatory models—that of the patient and that of the clinician.

This issue of how to conceptualize otherness in relation to suffering has been a key concern in anthropology. In writing on the mental health of migrants, anthropologists have shown that the characterization of culture as a catch-all in the

expression of mental disorders and in their treatment offers one way to depoliti-
cize distress and to avoid addressing the underlying socioeconomic inequalities
that produce it (Andoche 2001; Fassin 1999, 2000; Ong 1995; Rechtman 1995;
Santiago-Irizarry 2001; Watters 2001). Anthropologists have also been instrumental in documenting the importance of the relationship between cultural systems
and mental health and have underscored cross-cultural variations in constructions
of the self and of emotions (Csordas 1994; Desjarlais 1992; Jenkins 1991, 1996; Lutz
and White 1986; Shweder and Levine 1984; Shweder 1991, 2003). Anthropologists
have also been strong advocates for culturally sensitive therapeutic care (Kleinman
1980; Kleinman and Good 1985; Jenkins and Barrett 2004). However, the popularization of the notion of "cultural competency" in mental health initiatives, and
in public health generally, has led to essentializing understandings of the culture
concept and to its conflation with race and ethnicity (Santiago-Irizarry 2001).

Anthropologists have been critical of this trend. The critique (e.g., Carpenter-
Song, Schwallie, and Longhofer 2007) has concentrated on the tendency to characterize culture as fixed and static, the risk of perceiving cultural difference as a
form of social deviance, the unintentional blaming of the patient's culture as a barrier to effective treatment while ignoring structural features that may negatively
affect care, and the inability of some to recognize biomedicine—psychiatry in
particular—as a culturally constructed and historically evolving system. This last
critique led to important objections to alleged universal psychiatric disease categories as classified by the *Diagnostic and Statistical Manual of Mental Disorders*
(Gaines 1992) and to the manual's categorization of "culture-bound syndromes"
(Good and Good 2010; Guarnaccia 2003; Mezzich et al. 2009). Less often, with
the exception of psychiatry, anthropologists seek to propose clinically relevant and
practical recommendations (Carpenter-Song, Schwallie, and Longhofer 2007; see
also Guarnaccia 2003; Kirmayer 1997; Kleinman 1988; Kleinman and Benson
2006). Recent scholarship provides more nuanced analyses of how psychiatry, as
a discipline, responds to cultural diversity (Giordano 2014 ; Good et al. 2011;
Kirmayer 2012; Kirmayer, Guzder, and Rousseau 2014; Willen and Carpenter-Song
2013). Most of these analyses focus on the United States and Canada (with the
exceptions of Giordano 2014 on ethnopsychiatry in Italy and Kirmayer, Guzder,
and Rousseau 2014 on comparative perspectives between Canada and France or
Switzerland), which hold multiculturalism as foundational to their nations and
therefore directly acknowledge their populations' diversity. In this book, I focus
instead on the republican model of France and underscore how context is key in
responses to cultural diversity.

In the second part of the book, I introduce ethnographic data based on
referral narratives. Much has been written within literature in the social sciences and in psychology on the experiences of migrants. In contrast, I focus on
the professionals who assist migrants both within and beyond the clinical setting. I look at "the subtler moral positions" (Willen 2012, 805) that undergird

questions of entitlement and access to mental health care and that ultimately define professionals' senses of responsibility and ethics. In chapter 3, "Cultural and Linguistic Difference as Obstacles to Care," I try to capture a sense of how referring professionals, in particular, "translate" migrants' problems (Giordano 2014) through the language of both suffering and cultural difference. In turn, I assess the extent to which Centre Minkowska acts as a site where the essentialization of individuals—their reduction to an imagined cultural identity—is contested and the complexity of their life situations is restored, such as when staff members recognize these individuals' vulnerability and approach their cases from a structural vantage.

Referral narratives thus seemed to offer the best vantage point from which to observe intersections between medical and social management of immigrant populations and between state ideology and professional ethics. The common result of referral encounters I witnessed was the production of meta-discourse on the management of cultural difference in France. This type of discourse generates categorization dynamics based on "cultural repertoires" (Lamont 2000), which scholars consider to be a collection of social norms and values, often linguistically coded, with effects that tend to go unnoticed. It relates to what Dutch social scientist Philomena Essed called "everyday racism," which is "a process in which (a) socialized racist notions are integrated into meanings that make practices immediately definable and manageable, (b) practices with racist implications become in themselves familiar and repetitive, and (c) underlying racial and ethnic relations are actualized and reinforced through these routine or familiar practices in everyday situation" (1991, 52). Because this type of discourse is pervasive but often goes unnoticed by participants in the institutional referral process, I focused my research on the language of patient referrals. I pay particular attention to the language of difference as it is framed in the French context—where references to culture are perceived as inherently stigmatizing and anti-republican.

This "difficulty with naming" (la difficulté de dire, to borrow from Didier Fassin 2006) in contemporary France has a long history, and it is an apt example of cultural anxiety—the anxiety of multicultural France. The discourse of referring actors thus reveals unscripted perspectives that offer a glimpse into collective social reflections on identity, cultural difference, and the health treatment of migrant populations. In my research, I found that these types of discourse clearly illustrated that cultural difference is perceived by state agents in France as something that creates social *difficulties*, which in turn produce pathological situations. Such discourse is not necessarily articulated in stigmatizing terms but rather as benevolence toward migrants through a desire to help assuage their "difficulties."

In chapter 4, "Managing 'Migrant Youth,'" I focus on exploring the language of school referrals, which most directly conveys social understandings of a standard socialization model and of behavioral norms. I examine how definitions of normal behavior are articulated through school referrals related to negotiating plural identities for second-generation youth and to learning French and adjusting to a new environment for recently arrived youth. I argue that specialized mental health centers like Centre Minkowska represent loci where essentializing representations of migrants' cultural differences are projected and can be contested. I argue that school referrals to specialized mental health care unveil France's anxiety with sociodemographic change, the changing terms of "national identity," and the structural challenges of integration and settlement.

In the face of France's management of migrant populations, specialized mental health professionals contend with a particular ethical and structural dilemma: Do they abide by structural logics, which will lead them to "positively" differentiate so as to guarantee mental health care access to their migrant patients? Or do they contest these logics of stigmatization and exclusion at the risk of penalizing their patients and having them fall out of the system? Because of this dilemma, discourse within these institutions—as well as among interactions that take place in and around the clinic—about the referral of migrant patients are fraught with contradictions and inconsistencies. Specialized mental health experts routinely find themselves caught in double binds, wherein they are challenged to counter arbitrary or stigmatizing referrals. However, I suggest that specialized mental health centers, rather than contributing to the medicalization of migrants' cultural difference or to their social exclusion, constitute loci where relations of domination and inequalities are contested and, at times, challenged. This is where critical moral anthropology becomes relevant; it is an approach that offers an intermediate level for understanding the articulation between social context and the decisions and actions of social actors.

According to the moral economy perspective, not only do social agents apply state logics and policies but they constitute parts of the state (Fassin et al. 2013). This breaks with more traditional representations of the state as a monolithic whole that works for the greater good but primarily works in the interest of those in power. Critical moral anthropology holds that institutions are production sites for the state, located at the intersection of public space and professional habitus. They are constrained by a mission but also by social agents' own ethos (Fassin et al. 2013, 19). They are shaped by local and national contexts and are subject to change over time.

Although I draw on the critical moral anthropology framework in this book, I also find it limiting. It offers a narrow political frame that suggests—albeit rightfully—that initiatives for humanitarian, compassionate action and practice are often constrained by state regulations that reproduce existing social inequalities. As Miriam Ticktin (2011) has argued, the notion of suffering often constitutes the only legitimate space for migrants in what she calls "regimes of care." From that perspective, I would be bound to conclude that in relying on notions of suffering, specialized mental health care as a field creates a two-pronged system that indirectly produces and reproduces social boundaries between people who are deemed to belong (and are therefore suitable for mainstream health care) and those who are not—migrants and their children.

While I partly rely on this critical approach to investigate the double binds specialized mental health professionals experience in their work with migrants in France, I also explore what emerges from sites of contestation, such as Minkowska. I suggest that social actors—specifically referring state agents and specialized mental health professionals—are often cognizant of broad institutional norms, even though such norms exert powerful constraints on their agencies. Drawing on Paul Brodwin's (2013) notion of "everyday ethics," I identify clashes that occur between state agents' ideal framework of the clinic and the limits of the system within which it evolves or those that occur when the institution faces its own contradictions or double binds.

First, in chapter 5, "Enacting Cultural Competence," I analyze the institutional routines created at Centre Minkowska to try to standardize decisions so that a sense of coherence can be maintained in the face of deeply complex situations. What I call "complex situations" are those in which a person's suffering is deeply enmeshed with a "host of mutually reinforcing insults (ranging from the economic and political to the cultural and psychodynamic) that dispose [them] toward ill health" (Quesada, Hart, and Bourgois 2011). As it is construed at the center, the cultural competence approach—and the clinical medical anthropology model on which it rests—specifically means to address such complexity. I structure this chapter around the three pillars of cultural competence at Centre Minkowska: identifying explanatory models of suffering, decentering, and deliberating. Decentering refers to one's ability to take a step back from one's cultural frame of reference in order to make room for others. This process relies on reflexivity in the anthropological sense of the term: the ability to be critical of one's own social positioning and of its impact on one's interpretation of any given situation (Asad 1973; Clifford and Marcus 1986). Finally, deliberating relies on the creation of a safe space to enable people to share not only information and knowledge but also affect in their attempts to make sense of complex situations. This way of deliberating is enacted through MEDIACOR meetings. Ultimately, the cultural competence approach and the processes it relies on *should* enable professionals—regardless of their training *and*, importantly, of their cultural identity—to both maintain a sense of coherence and experience empathy in the face of the most complex, radically foreign situations. It allows professionals to manage uncertainty and to accept situations in which they may find themselves in a position of "not-knowing" (Guzder and Rousseau 2013).

In chapter 6, "Psychotherapy at the Borderland," I explore how staff at Minkowska in particular have adapted their clinical practice to accommodate situations "at the borderland"—that is, situations in which social issues are predominant and hinder psychotherapeutic work. I refer here to situations of extreme precarity, when patients' uncertainties about obtaining legal status or accessing basic needs, such as a place to sleep or food to eat, makes time chatting with a psychotherapist almost irrelevant. This chapter thus highlights the meaning of "structural vulnerability" in the clinical context. A critical question I raise in this context is whether Centre Minkowska is instrumentalized by the state as a stop-gap for excluded migrant populations. I highlight MEDIACOR meetings as opportunities to evaluate how Minkowska professionals use the cultural compe-tence approach, based on clinical medical anthropology, to "lean into the situation and search for a way through it" (Brodwin 2013, 10) in order to endorse senti-ments of responsibility and care. I investigate how ruptures between professionals' ideals and system logics fuel feelings of frustration, provide an impetus for staff members to take responsibility and action, and differentially affect experts accord-ing to their professional statuses and experiences. I suggest MEDIACOR offers a space of ethical deliberations where these affective logics of work, as I call them, are integrated and where interstices of caregiving and the contestation of stigma-tizing referrals can be identified.

In chapter 7, "Beyond Anxieties: Praxis," I reflect on what emerges from the clinical medical anthropology and the related cultural competence approaches practiced at Minkowska. What actions are produced from that clinical experience that may lead to new forms of inclusion for migrants? What actions lead to new ways of construing our understandings of what is human within the field of health care? I argue that while the contradictions and double binds specialized mental health professionals face are anxiety producing, they also offer fertile ground for resistance and for ethical response. In this book, I show how such anxieties—and responses to them—may not necessarily redefine the structuring contours of our political-economic system and the health care institutions located within it but may gradually help challenge them.

I have been tempted to conclude that Minkowska limits its practical challenge to the structural misrecognition (Taylor 1994) of migrants in France through its persistence in occupying an institutionally ambiguous space. However, I critically assess and discuss the practical impacts of Centre Minkowska—and the cultural competence approach more broadly—on the contemporary management of migrants in France and on migrants' structural vulnerability. I elaborate how MEDIACOR's reflexive and systemic approach offers a promising institutional framework for dealing with the complexities of human behavior in health care while also assuming the urgent need for service provision. Ultimately, I suggest that the transcultural clinic—and other borderland institutions like it—constitutes a laboratory where people may experiment with and practice a politics of hospi-tality. It is a place where people's experiences provide lessons for social justice and for improved caregiving practices—not only for migrants but for those who find themselves in situations of extreme vulnerability.

A DAY AT CENTRE
MINKOWSKA

It is a fine Parisian morning in the fall of 2018, and I am on my way to work at Centre Minkowska. I walk down l'avenue de Clichy and turn left onto rue Jacquemont, a small street where the Centre is located in a compact three-story building. Other than a couple of restaurants toward the end, most structures on the street are residential. I recently realized that Victor Jacquemont was a famous French botanist and geologist who traveled the world by sea during the 1820s for research and spoke against the slavery practiced in the colonies at the time. I found it an amusing coincidence that the Centre Minkowska, which caters to migrants from across the world and supports their rights generally and their access to health care in particular, is located on a street named after a world traveler who shared similar values. I walk up the building's narrow staircase to the third floor, which opens onto a small landing at the very top of the building. Often when I come to work in the morning, the center has not yet opened, and I pass patients who sit on the stairs, waiting. In the summer, when the weather warms, this landing feels like a steam room; it is exposed to direct skylight through its large glass windows and roof.

As I enter the center, I greet the secretaries who sit at a desk facing the entry-way. I then head directly to my office, which is located to the left of the entrance. After leaving my coat and purse in the office, which I share with my two colleagues, Laetitia and Christine, I join the center's other staff members in the cafeteria room, where we chat for about twenty minutes over coffee or tea. There are usually six or seven of us who work full time at the center: Marie-Jo, Christophe, Laetitia, Christine, Verthançia, and me. Christophe is Centre Minkowska's director, Marie-Jo is its joint director, and Verthançia is its social worker. Laetitia and Christine both work for the center's professional training department. Depending on the day, other staff members might join us, including attending psychiatrists such as Dr. Cheref or Dr. Carlin and psychologists such as Daria. We often talk about the news, our next vacation destination, or our experiences with our children or grandchildren. At times, colleagues bring *viennoiseries*, or homemade cakes.

The atmosphere at Centre Minkowska is familial. The team of full-time professionals and part-time clinicians is relatively small, and as we have worked together
for a long time, we have grown to know one another well. Generally, I address
all my colleagues—including those higher in the center's hierarchy—using the
French pronoun *tu*. This is not very common in French professional contexts,
where the formal pronoun *vous* would be more appropriate. Laetitia, who was
recently hired as a development officer for the professional training department,
often notes how shocked she was when she first witnessed the level of familiarity here and was invited for drinks at a colleague's home just a few months after
arriving. Of course, as with families, such closeness can have a downside; staff
members sometimes become involved in disagreements or conflicts where this
familiarity impedes professional interaction.

Following our coffee break, Marie-Jo asks me if I will follow her to her office;
she has something she wants to discuss. Marie-Jo is in her early seventies, but she
looks much younger. She is a blond, blue-eyed, midsize woman, with strong
energy and an assertive streak. She is the first person I met when I introduced
myself at the center in 2007 as a doctoral student. At the time, she made a strong
impression on me, and I was a bit intimidated by her. Hired in 1982, she is currently Centre Minkowska's longest-working staff member. Her first job at the
center was as a social worker, at a time when the center was organized around
geolinguistic departments; Marie-Jo was in charge of the departments that
catered to Portuguese-speaking people and to those from African countries. For
Marie-Jo, working at Centre Minkowska was an opportunity to combine her
interest in community psychiatry with her desire to work for the French branch
of the Social Service for Support to Emigrants (SSAE).

In my experience, Marie-Jo is the kind of person who likes to take the initiative whenever she can, and this trait is prominent throughout her history: she
found herself increasingly taking leadership roles at the center and created a professional training service in 1986, which she continues to direct today. During her
graduate studies in social work, she produced a thesis on legal trials that occurred
around the issue of female genital cutting (FGC) in France. For the past thirty
years, she has interacted with women who have undergone FGC and who have
sought clitoral reconstructive surgery—or women who are seen at the center in
the context of related therapy. When working with women who plan a surgical
intervention, Marie-Jo collaborates with a Parisian-based hospital unit, and she
attends the unit's staff meetings on a monthly basis. She recently published a book
on that clinical experience (Bourdin 2013). She also has a long history of visiting
and working in Senegal. Her office—the largest at the center—is decorated with
photos and souvenirs from her trips to Senegal and to other countries in West
Africa, including Mali and Benin.

On this particular day, Marie-Jo wants to debrief me about a face-to-face experience she had had in her office with a traditional cutter. She says, "Can you

imagine? I'm the first to talk about the importance of decentering in transcultural situations, and there I was, with a traditional cutter in front of me! I felt the anger rise within me as I understood what was going on. I did all I could to not make it obvious, but I think it showed through in my facial expression and tone of voice." The lady who had come to her office the day before, whom we'll call Mrs. P, was a Yoruba-speaking asylum seeker from Nigeria who also spoke limited English. Because she complained of major sleep disorders and nightmares, she had been referred to Centre Minkowska by the educator at her housing residence. The referring letter mentioned that she had undergone FGC but that her request for help was rather vague. It was with this minimal amount of information that Marie-Jo had met Mrs. P. In a way, this situation typifies the complicated referral requests we encounter at the center: such requests often originate with a wide array of institutional actors outside the mental health field, and the referral relevance often has to be made intelligible by the professionals at Minkowska. It can sometimes feel like a guessing game. This is one of the main reasons why MEDIACOR, the referral-screening unit, was created in 2009.

Marie-Jo continues to explain how, during the first evaluation meeting with two English-speaking colleagues, communication was so limited that Mrs. P had to sometimes mime her conversational responses. At one point, she even stood up from her chair, sat on the ground, spread her legs, and, pointing to her genitals, mimicked a scissoring gesture. Marie-Jo says, "So I immediately thought she had been excised and came to France to protect her daughter." And so Marie-Jo scheduled a second appointment for Mrs. P with a professional Yoruba interpreter. It was during that second meeting that Mrs. P explained that she was a professional cutter and had been trained by her own mother. She had been chosen by the oracle to train other women and to encourage mothers to excise their daughters. But, she noted, she started questioning her mission when a few of the girls on whom she had worked died after hemorrhagic complications or tetanus. Marie-Jo continues: "I was stunned! I surprised myself [by] staring at her hands, wondering how many girls she had mutilated."

Later on, with the help of the interpreter, Marie-Jo understood that the reason Mrs. P decided to stop excising girls was out of love for her husband, who was morally against the practice. As she rallied her husband's clan, her own family threatened her and her husband for questioning the oracle. After her husband was reported missing, she decided to flee to France with her daughter. It took some time for Marie-Jo to be able to "decenter" and to agree to continue seeing this woman—a woman who had actively engaged in a practice Marie-Jo had denounced for so long.

Decentering is a critical practice at Centre Minkowska, and it is a concept I will unpack throughout this ethnography. It is a work of posture—an ability to step back from one's representations and, at times, from one's emotions related to the judgment (often negative) of things foreign or unknown. This is a key concept in the transcultural clinic, and it is related to the process of transference active in the patient-clinician dyad. In psychoanalytic theory, transference refers to the process by which the unconscious desires of the analysand become actual and are projected (transferred) onto the person of the analyst (Freud [1949] 1989). Transference affects both participants in the therapeutic setting. "Counter-transference" refers specifically to an analyst's unconscious projection onto the analysand. The ability for the analyst—or clinician—to identify the transferential process at work is itself a clinical tool. It can be likened to the process of reflexivity as an anthropological (and broader social science) method—that is, the anthropologist's efforts to identify the effect of his or her presence in the field and the ability to distantiate him- or herself from his or her worldview in order to be as open as possible to the worldviews of others. In other words, it is the very process through which empathy is enabled in a context where cultural representations and moral values are likely to differ.

As we will explore in this ethnography, the work of decentering is central to Centre Minkowska's cultural competence approach, and it constitutes the very basis of what staff members consider hospitable practices. It is a logic of caregiving that integrates uncertainty in the management of cultural difference or structural complexity and thus allows professionals to move beyond anxieties triggered by complex situations.

* * *

After a lunch break, we all congregate again in the cafeteria room. Consultations resume at 2:00 P.M., and we do not spend as much time having coffee and chatting as we tend to do in the mornings. Dr. Rachid Bennegadi arrives. He is a tall, balding man with sparse gray hair, and like Marie-Jo, he is in his early seventies. On all days except Friday, Dr. Bennegadi works at the center only during the afternoons. In the mornings, he maintains a private practice located near Gare du Nord. When he arrives, he often takes time to stop for coffee and to greet everyone. He also regularly monopolizes any conversation and launches into discussions of literature and the arts. For example, he will start by voicing his admiration for Woody Allen and finish with a summary of Antonio Damasio's latest book. His undeniable oratory skills tend to capture everyone's attention. He also has a great sense of humor and is known for his puns. From what I have seen, many interns who come to Minkowska appear quite intimidated by him. I suspect I owe him, in part, for my position at Centre Minkowska: as the "thinking head" behind the implementation of a clinical medical anthropology approach, he advocated for having an anthropologist on staff, even though no room for that position existed in the work convention that regulates the institution. In our conversations, he has told me that throughout his career, he has fought to avoid being the designated Arab who gets offered positions to play politics of representations. I believe his sense of humor partly developed as a defense mechanism to cope with the innumerable stigmatizing situations in which he has found himself over the years. Undoubtedly, his personal experience also deeply nourished his reflections on the meaning of transcultural care and his quest for a more nuanced and relevant concept of culture within contemporary mental health.

This day, Dr. Bennegadi invites me to attend a consultation with a five-year-old autistic child, Lofti, who is accompanied by his mother. Lofti was referred to Dr. Bennegadi directly by a general practitioner who has referred Arab-speaking patients from Maghreb to the center in the past. Lofti's parents are from Algeria. In this case, the mother speaks French, and she speaks both French and Arabic with Lofti. This is Dr. Bennegadi's initial meeting with Lofti and his mother. First, he spends some time interacting with Lofti. Lofti is extremely agitated. He barely speaks, and the words he pronounces are hardly understandable. Dr. Bennegadi manages to get him to focus for a few minutes on a game that consists of clapping hands, but Lofti quickly loses interest and returns to sit near his mother. Dr. Bennegadi tries to interest him in drawing something, but Lofti eventually loses patience, puts his hands over his ears, and produces a deep, throaty growl to express his discontent. I manage to gain Lofti's attention by drawing myself on the sheet of paper Dr. Bennegadi gave him. Meanwhile, Dr. Bennegadi speaks with Lofti's mother about the boy's situation, as well as about her experience at home. The two switch back and forth between French and Arabic. I notice they switch to Arabic when they refer to family members' representations of Lofti's disorder or when they discuss strategies, such as spanking, that are deployed at home to manage his clastic behavior (unintentional bursts of aggressiveness or violence).

From their interaction, it sounds to me as though Lofti is closely monitored by various institutions and has been seen by many professionals. After Lofti and his mother leave the office, I ask Dr. Bennegadi why Lofti was referred to Minkowska, considering that he has been in care since he was eight months old and currently sees both a pediatrician and a child psychiatrist on a regular basis at the hospital. Dr. Bennegadi hypothesizes that Lofti's general practitioner most likely wanted to check on the mother and to investigate how the family was coping with the situation. In this session, Dr. Bennegadi acts as both a psychiatrist who evaluates the situation and a cultural mediator who relies on language to help Lofti's mother feel comfortable speaking about the family's experience of his situation. For example, she spoke about how her mother-in-law constantly advises her what to do or not to do with the child. She also talked about her husband's temptation to use spanking as a way to calm Lofti down during his fits.

Cultural and linguistic familiarity, such as the one that exists between Dr. Bennegadi and this mother, are elements that can favorably affect the therapeutic relationship and outcome. In fact, ideas about such familiarity are often the very motives that compel other state agents to refer patients to Centre Minkowska. However, the cultural competence approach, as practiced at the center, avoids drawing this direct equation between cultural expertise—that of the clinician with respect to his or her cultural and linguistic background—and transcultural clinical practice. Rather, cultural competence is evaluated through the therapist's ability to decenter from his or her own cultural representations and to relate to the patient's representations so that psychopathological elements may be identified and a diagnosis made. Beyond that, cultural competence refers to the clinician's ability to consider broader social determinants that may affect both the patient's distress or the therapy itself—and his or her ability to act on it in the clinic. Of course, the ability to communicate is paramount, and in a transcultural setting, if patient and clinician do not share the same language, this approach remains irrelevant. As a result, other institutional actors usually refer Arabic-speaking Maghreb patients to Dr. Bennegadi or other clinicians at the center who speak Arabic. However, if a patient's language is not spoken by any clinician at the center, a common language can usually be found. For example, I speak English and have interacted with several patients from English-speaking sub-Saharan African countries, such as Nigeria and Uganda. When these two options cannot be met, the center resorts to professional interpreters, as illustrated in the situation with Marie-Jo's patient, Mrs. P.

From this perspective, cultural competence—with training and practice—lies within reach of every professional. From a theoretical perspective, this sounds logical. However, in practice, it creates ambiguities—both on the part of referring agents and on the part of clinicians themselves—about what, exactly, constitutes the center's expertise. If members of any mental health institution who are trained in cultural competence are as able as we are to work with professional interpreters and with differing cultural representations of mental suffering, then what need is there for an expert institution such as Centre Minkowska? As we will see throughout this ethnography, such questions are closely linked to the French ideological context and its management of cultural difference. They are also linked to broader structural logics that lead the center to act as a stopgap for excluded populations and to face particular ethical dilemmas, or "double binds," as I call them in this book.

* * *

At 4:00 P.M., it is now time for me to attend our referral meeting: MEDIACOR. The room is packed, and there are barely enough seats for all of us to attend. As the head of this screening unit, Marie-Jo is there—as she always is. Both psychiatrists, Dr. Bennegadi and Dr. Cheref, are present. Dr. Cheref is a tall and slender man in his mid-fifties. He is a jovial person but has a very different personality than Dr. Bennegadi. While he also takes time to teach interns during these meetings, he is less inclined than Dr. Bennegadi to discuss theory or ethics at length. Dr. Cheref is a more straight-to-the-point, practical thinker, and he rarely cuts corners when he speaks. At times, I find his handling of clinical cases a bit abrupt. In a sense, his and Dr. Bennegadi's personalities are complementary in their approaches to the center's work.

On this day, MEDIACOR receives a guest named Dr. Melissa Dominicé Dao. She is a physician who heads the cultural consultation unit at a university hospital in Geneva (Dominicé Dao et al. 2018) and who gives a yearly lecture on her experience to professionals in Minkowska's continuing education program. Marie-Jo, Daria Rostirolla (an Italian psychologist and medical anthropologist), six therapists in training (TEFs, *thérapeutes en formation*), and I are discussing the referral of a Russian-speaking Chechen man in need of psychiatric care. Unfortunately, Minkowska does not have a Russian-speaking psychiatrist. Because the person who referred the man did so using a logic based only on linguistic competence, our discussion revolves around whose responsibility it is to work with an interpreter—Centre Minkowska or the referring district mental health center (CMP). We also discuss the relevance of transcultural care within the broader French public health landscape.

Considering that Minkowska has a multilingual team, the logic behind referring on the basis of language could be considered legitimate. However, we discuss two points that undermine this. First, state agents systematically refer nonfrancophone patients without trying to work with interpreters at all—not even to try to assess the actual *need* for a mental health follow-up. Second, not all clinicians at Minkowska speak all requested languages. In those cases, the center must rely on interpreters, even though it usually has no greater financial means than the referring institution. The following exchange, a continuation of this discussion of the Chechen migrant, attests to this dilemma:

DR. CHEREF (DR. C): So the language obstacle is probably going to make follow-up difficult.

MARIE-JO (MJ): And CMPs do not want to work with interpreters.

DR. BENNEGADI (DR. B): And that's often the alibi for the cultural to come up.

DR. DOMINICÉ DAO (DR. DD): Yes, it's the problem of the traditional health-care system; it does not work with interpreters.

MJ: Well, some do, but very few.

DR. C: Very few.

DR. B: So, the linguistic competence?

TEF: Russian.

DR. B: So, Russian-speaking Chechen?

DR. C: He's forty-six, so he went to a Russian school . . .

. . .

MJ: I would simply say that we have no Russian-speaking psychiatrist, period.

DR. B: And he doesn't speak French?

MJ: Limited French.

DR. B: I don't know, who has a particular opinion on this? Go ahead! What can we do to help him? We have a referral that's mediatized by colleagues … so maybe that's not all there is to it.

MJ: Yes … I would respond that we don't have a Russian-speaking psychiatrist and that they can refer him to a CMP with an interpreter.

DARIA (D): And in our network, we don't have anybody?

DR. B: No, we don't. Only in the private sector.

MJ: They won't be able to pay for it.

DR. B: I think it's safe and very professional at once to tell them [referring professionals]: "Listen, we are going to do what you can do yourself [meaning: working with an interpreter]; we won't do more." And maintain a coherence in the follow-up, by keeping it within the *Secteur*.

MJ: Yes, proximity! [Patient's residence] is far away [from the center]!

This extended, hesitant deliberation between six people about whether the center should take over the situation—and thus assume responsibility for financing interpreter services ourselves—is indicative of the deep, consistent concern Minkowska staff exhibit regarding the consequences of our decisions. Each new situation challenges our sense of responsibility once we learn of it: What will become of the patient if we decline this referral? Can we ensure there will be appropriate follow-up care elsewhere? This concern about responsibility emerges regularly as an ethical dilemma in discussions and is evidenced in the following conversation:

DR. B: So, who here thinks that we are shirking our responsibilities? Come on, we must consider all options here.

. . .

D: I don't think we are shirking our responsibilities. We are often overwhelmed by referrals that go beyond our framework and our limits, so I find it relevant not to put a colleague in a potentially dangerous situation, and at the same time, I think there are maybe preconceived ideas about the fact that he cannot be seen by a *Secteur* psychiatrist.

MJ: No, I think we can very well say …

DR. B: No, it's important to hear about the argument, to understand why we say yes, why we say no, why we say maybe.

. . .

DR. C: Health-care access in the private sector is impossible—

DR. B: No, that's not the issue. We are between us. We are being considered as an associative institution that comes in to fill a gap, or there's no gap, just the fact that colleagues don't allow themselves to work with an interpreter.

MJ: Exactly.

. . .

DR. C: In my opinion, they are not trying to avoid the situation. They ask for our advice: "You probably have a Russian-speaking psychiatrist, you may be able to take this patient."

DR. B: . . . We must put in that the point is also to keep a territorial coherence; that's how we need to explain it, so that they understand that it's not a rejection. And always with the formula at the end: "We remain at your disposal in the event that . . . etc." Which is absolutely deontological. Imagine they only need an evaluation, then we know that the patient will be seen; we do the job on the side, and we send the information back. It remains public health. It's very complicated to work on public health when we receive such referrals because we have a tendency to find ourselves rejecting certain requests. That's not what we do. MEDIACOR doesn't function that way. It's not about rejecting but about understanding why we say no. And why we refer to others.

MJ: Dr. S will do the mail.

DR. B: In Russian, obviously! (*Laughs.*)

Humorous interjections such as this one happen recurrently during MEDIACOR meetings. In her ethnography of American psychiatric clients, American anthropologist Sue Estroff notes how the use of humor by clinical staff often serves to channel hostility or frustration and helps release tension in the face of difficult situations or bizarre behavior (1985, 28–29). This is certainly relevant in the MEDIACOR context, particularly when it comes to discussing heavy situations or, as in the case here, identifying arguments about why a patient cannot be received at the center.

A third situation we discuss at MEDIACOR this day echoes the first; it concerns a Bengali-speaking migrant referred to Minkowska on the basis of language obstacles. Contrary to the first situation, the team decides to use an interpreter to carry out an evaluation with this migrant. This is partly because several other Bengali-speaking migrants had been referred to Minkowska in the previous few days, and the team decides that one interpreter could be mobilized for an entire morning of evaluation sessions with Dr. Cheref. Although the financial argument is not verbalized in the following exchange, it is a concern that generally colors decisions at Minkowska and triggers tense debates. At the moment I detail in the following exchange, Dr. Dominicé Dao decides to address the apparent contradiction between taking a Bengali-speaking migrant—when there was no Bengali-speaking therapist on staff—and refusing the Russian-speaking migrant:

DR. DD: And the difference with the first person from Chechnya is that this person already receives care from a mental health-care professional, is that the difference? . . . So, finally, we accept . . . sorry, I'm playing troublemaker here, but in the end, we accept the Bengali-speaking person, not the Russian-speaking one?

DR. B: Because the referral and the issue are different . . . we take into account all elements: those who have possibilities, those who do not, the acuity of problems at stake, and the competence that we have. We are obligated to take all of this into account.

MJ: And in this last case, we are going to make an evaluation, which does not mean that there will be a follow-up. We are going to make an evaluation to potentially refer him somewhere else.

TEF: The first patient had the advantage to be connected to a CMP through his children.

MJ: And there's already a local follow-up.

DR. B: We try to validate the coherence of the system itself, without using the system as a scapegoat, which would be ridiculous. We are the first here to fight against the scapegoating of people, so if we start saying, "Oh, colleagues can't do their jobs," we always avoided that, it's useless to assign this responsibility to someone. What do we do for this person? The best we can do, and we are *able to* do—we are careful not to turn into megalomaniacs and say, "We accept, we accept, we accept." That's not an intelligible attitude. In public health, that doesn't make sense. We accept, and above all, we all learned here to explain why we accept. We provide arguments, and we debate between us to decide whether it makes sense or not. [emphasis in original]

What these exchanges capture are the main challenges that staff at Minkowska face during negotiations around referrals—the specifics of which will be the object of following chapters. Although Dr. Bennegadi plays it down in his response to Dr. Dominicé Dao, many patients are referred to Minkowska due to inadequacies in the broader social services and health-care systems. The complex contours of migrants' personal and social circumstances challenge referring state agents, who in turn use the notion of culture or use language barriers to justify their decisions to refer migrants to other professionals—thereby passing responsibility to someone else down the line. To some extent, irritation and futility seem to be an inevitable part of staff experience at places like Centre Minkowska; such feelings creep into staff members' reactions as they analyze and identify the instrumental logics behind state agents' referrals of migrant patients. But MEDIACOR offers a distanced, deliberative space where staff members' affective experiences have room for broader expression:

DR. B: The trap we fell in at MEDIACOR at the beginning consisted in a certain form of irritation, a form of unconscious aggressiveness towards people who refer to us. We realized one thing, which is that some referrals are so stigmatizing, that we feel stigmatized by the fact that we are considered as culture specialists. We are *not* culture specialists. We are specialists of patient care, within which cultural representations appear. And that is something which is not natural for the human psychic functioning.

DR. DD: We felt the same. And with my colleagues, we wondered whether we did not stigmatize patients by the very fact of accepting them. And our choice was to do it regardless, and to unpack things.

DR. B: That's the ethical part!

DR. DD: And to say, indeed, the patient does not speak the same language, indeed, a number of values are different, but there's also the fact that he is homeless, that he experienced violence, that he was rejected from his asylum request, and we unpack things.

DR. B: And that's exactly what we do, by getting back to people, to show them we are not fooled by the enormity of the referral, and that at the same time, we don't accuse anyone. It's very complicated to respond. Very complicated.

ME: That's why there's no systematic response from one situation to another. In evaluations, there are different forms of complexity.

DR. B: Most important is to learn to argue why we accept or why not. It makes the rationale more intelligible.

MEDIACOR meetings amount to intense ethical deliberation in response to migrant patients' situations, which are complex and inherently singular. As I show in later chapters, every patient has a different history, set of social relationships, economic circumstances, and other entanglements that come together in unique ways that must be unpacked on a case-by-case basis. As such, what constitutes a referral considered legitimate by Centre Minkowska's staff, one that actually benefits from the staff's expertise, can never be determined through normative or standardized means.

While MEDIACOR staff rely on clinical medical anthropology and cultural competence frameworks to help them identify a comprehensive set of dimensions that affect the referral, they also wrestle with different rationales when analyzing each situation. Different points of view, which express both professional ethics and personal affect, are considered during deliberations. At the end of this collaborative process, there is no right or wrong answer. Rather, there is an answer whose rationale has been made "more intelligible." Importantly, this process enables the expression of and deliberation on ambiguous positions, which are often less tolerated in other medical spaces, such as hospitals and CMPs. As Dr. Bennegadi commented that same day, "Instead of making the patient more schizophrenic than necessary, we accept that we'll have to become a little schizophrenic to avoid disadvantaging the patient. So, at times we are in very ambiguous, borderline positions." In a sense, MEDIACOR helps staff members at Minkowska manage ethical anxieties that arise from the context in which they operate. Ultimately, I suggest that staff members prioritize the logics of caregiving.

Dr. Dominice Dao expresses this in her reaction to the stigmatizing logics that underpin referrals to her Geneva-based cultural consultation service: she provides care, regardless, and helps referring agents unpack individual situations. Does her choice, or the choices of staff at MEDIACOR, support a stigmatizing order? On the contrary, I would argue that their efforts to resist the cultural and linguistic categories used by state agents to frame "migrant suffering," and to critically reflect on appropriate clinical responses to potentially stigmatizing referrals, *challenge* the ways in which referrals to specialized mental health centers act as a regulative force in the lives of migrants.

As I will show in this ethnography, the MEDIACOR unit at Centre Minkowska has become the absolute pulse of the institution and the site of both the production and enactment of its expertise. Here, professionals "decenter"—that is, take a step back—from their clinical activities and constantly reformulate their professional goals and ethics in relation to the center's overarching mission of integrating migrants through health care. It has also become a pedagogical and social setting; increasing numbers of psychologists, psychiatrists, and psychotherapists in training attend the meetings to learn how to analyze referrals and tentatively formulate diagnoses. Most acutely, it highlights the articulations—through staff members' reflexivity about the referral process—between shared cultural representations of migrant individuals and their lifestyles, which are often intangible, and their materialization and circulation through institutional reports. The work done by staff members at MEDIACOR also makes visible different steps that occur in the process of making referrals, including their evaluation and negotiation within specialized mental health centers.

PART I

THE CONTEXT

In the first part of this book, I describe the context in which specialized mental health care emerged. To do so, I address the evolution of scientific discourse in the management of racial and cultural difference in mental health initiatives in the French colonies and in France. In the context of migration to France, I examine how migrant subjectivities are socially constructed; travel through time; and are reproduced, contested, or negotiated through the scientific discourse of specialized mental health.

I then situate Centre Minkowska within this field of specialized mental health care. I describe how the center developed and gained legitimacy within the field, and the tensions it met in the process. I focus on how France's ideological context and the recent managerial policies in health care underpinned Centre Minkowska's choice of a medical anthropology approach to mental health care as a way to destigmatize the patient-clinician encounter and to better evaluate clinical practice through public health standards.

1 · A GENEALOGY OF "MIGRANT SUFFERING"

The figure of the *migrant* has dominated the global collective imaginary in the twenty-first century (Nail 2015). Specific social representations of migrants have evolved in different contexts at different times: the labor migrant, asylum seeker, refugee, *sans-papiers*, unaccompanied minor. For migrants in general, social legitimacy is often evaluated institutionally and popularly by their cause of displacement—was it voluntary or involuntary? Voluntary migration is often perceived as less legitimate on the grounds that migrants may be searching for economic opportunity; this can activate social anxieties over limited resources in host countries. An exception is the "expatriates" category—a form of voluntary migration, often motivated by economic opportunity, but interestingly never labeled as migration. Moral demarcations around migration are fluid, and even the politics of hospitality in any given place or time can be contradictory.

The politics of migration in France are the embodiment of such contradiction, and social debates around the right to health care provide lively discussions about notions of integration and belonging (Larchanché 2012; Sargent and Larchanché 2009; Ticktin 2011). For example, shortly before his election as president in 2017, Emmanuel Macron declared in an interview that France was not confronted with "a wave of immigration" as portrayed by the media, that "the immigration issue should not worry the French population," and that "immigration is constitutive of the world we live in . . . [and] can even be an opportunity from an economic, cultural and social perspective" (Casadesus 2017, my translation). Shortly thereafter, his appointed interior minister, Gérard Collomb, announced that the necessary regulation of migration entailed a clear distinction between refugees and economic migrants: "Our policy must combine efficiency and generosity. We welcome those who flee wars and persecutions, but we distinguish refugees from those whose migration obeys other motivations, including economic ones" (*Le Monde* 2017, my translation). Beyond refugees, whose suffering and vulnerability are perceived as legitimate, it appears from Collomb's words that other migrants are unwelcome. Representations like these, largely disseminated through media and political rhetoric, rarely address the survival logics forcing perceived voluntary migrants to leave their homes in the midst of structural violence and economic inequality. The global war on terror has further complicated the dynamic by raising suspicion even about refugees.

Simultaneously, we are bombarded with media images of migration-related suffering: people fleeing brutality in war-torn zones, being rescued from the Mediterranean Sea, experiencing inhumane living conditions in cramped French encampments, or facing new forms of slavery in Libya. These images "engage in emotional and political work, producing sympathy and empathy, as well as fear and othering" (Holmes and Castaneda 2016, 17). Images of suffering in places far away can be particularly effective at instilling sympathy (Boltanski 1999), particularly when that suffering concerns children. This was illustrated through the case of Alan Kurdi, a three-year-old Syrian boy of Kurdish ethnic background who died on a beach in Turkey in 2015 and was photographed lying facedown in the sand. The photograph of Kurdi's body triggered profound emotional responses, expressed through social media across the globe. Images of suffering at home, however, can trigger uneasiness. Indeed, reports of appalling life conditions in encampments like Calais and Grande-Synthe in northern France, or the Stalingrad neighborhood in Paris, are unlikely to cause a similar outpouring of communal sympathy, even though children Alan Kurdi's age or younger suffer intensely from infectious pathologies in these areas (*L'Express* 2015).

When you hear the phrase "migrant suffering," you may presume that the acknowledgment of suffering itself is indicative of compassion or sympathy, meaning that suffering individuals are deserving of care and attention. But in relation to migrants in France, there are clear hierarchies of suffering, and the moral judgments that underpin them are shaped by complex interactions between local *"cultural representations, collective processes,* and *subjectivity,* interactions that are in turn shaped by large-scale changes in political economy, politics, and culture" (Kleinman 1998, 373). Moral experience, then, possesses both a locality and a genealogy that can be traced.

In this chapter, I trace the evolution of the notion of "migrant suffering" as a moral experience in France. A specialized form of mental health support directed at migrants developed in France in the aftermath of World War II. Fassin and Rechtman (2009, 226) argue that the genesis of this approach to mental health care for migrants occurred at the transition between two historical stages, each characterized by singular representations of cultural difference: the colonial era, with its image of the indigenous colonized "other," and the postcolonial period, with the figure of the migrant foreigner in search of employment or asylum. Mental health practitioners interested in the mental health of migrants found themselves caught between two psychopathological paradigms: the culturalist model of colonial psychiatry—imbued by racist interpretations of cultural personality types and ultimately concerned more with political order than psychopathology—and the universalist model of the French health-care system, which rejects the idea that migrants require "specialized" treatment. What structural context produced the necessary conditions for the emergence of a specialized field of mental health focused specifically on figures of alterity? What are the contemporary representations of cultural others that animated the growth of this field? In answering these questions, I begin to explore a genealogy of the management of otherness in French health care and the types of institutional and individual anxieties produced in the process.

COLONIAL LEGACIES: PATHOLOGIZING RACIAL AND CULTURAL DIFFERENCE

Theories of human behavior surrounding French psychiatric practice from the 1870s to the 1950s were racially biased and influenced by debates among anthropologists as well as psychiatrists. Colonial psychiatry generated discussion among both clinicians and scholars about the influence of race on mind and behavior, questions of cultural difference, and the political evolution of colonial subjects. As British historian Megan Vaughan (2007) notes, colonial psychiatry provided a scientific language with which to frame dilemmas encountered by colonial administrations. Alongside anthropologists, psychiatrists elaborated theories of "acculturation," "culture contact," and the "educability" of people from African countries. Such theories were politically relevant and addressed "the question of whether and when increasingly 'detribalized' Africans would ever be ready to govern themselves" (Vaughan 2007, 8). Both anthropology and psychiatry provided negative answers to this question and encouraged the pursuit of colonial management (Vaughan 2007).

In some colonial psychiatric theories, "culture" was merely a more acceptable term for "race." While anthropologists concentrated on changes at the level of "tribal" entities, psychiatrists offered a distinct medico-psychological approach, which located the detrimental effect of "culture contact" within individual personality and psyche. The basis for this approach was the notion of biological difference and its influence on relationships between race and psychopathology. Biological racism provided a scientific basis for the ideological opposition between "civilized" (European) and "primitive" mentalities (Vaughan 2007, 24).

The Case of the Algiers School: Colonial Psychiatry in the French Colony

In his exhaustive account of the practice of psychiatry in colonial North Africa, medical historian Richard Keller (2007) accounts for colonial psychiatrists' fascination with the relationship between psychology and culture. In the so-called primitive mind of the colonized, many of these psychiatrists found elements of a primordial, universal human subjectivity and considered this proof of the existence of an essential psychic unity. Yet psychiatrists working in colonial North

Africa sought to demonstrate a clear separation between the minds of Europeans and those of North Africans based on bodies and traditions. They followed the lead of French psychiatrist Antoine Porot, who in his 1918 publication "Notes de psychiatrie musulmane" (Notes on Muslim psychiatry) presented the scientific bases for such psychic demarcation, from which the Algiers School emerged. Difference between Europeans and North Africans existed, Porot's followers argued, and this was exacerbated by the colonial encounter, which thrust primitive people into an alienating modern environment. Drawing on the legacy of psychological anthropologists, physicians, and racial biologists of the time, their work produced a new science of colonial psychiatry with pragmatic applications for judicial, social, and military institutions. At the time, French psychiatrists characterized North African Muslim populations as inferior to civilized Europeans "by documenting the Maghrebian's temperamental violence, fatalism, superstitions, and mental debilitation" (Keller 2007, 123).

This type of colonial psychiatry constituted a form of "military organism" (Keller 2007, 123), articulated around the language of battle and deployed in the service of colonial power to tame unruly indigenous populations and shape debates over law enforcement and immigration. According to Keller, the outbreak of war in 1914 and the presence of colonial subjects in the infantry provided psychiatrists with the opportunity to study indigenous populations under stress and draw conclusions on racial and cultural influences on psychopathology. French psychiatrists Antoine Porot and Angelo Hesnard (1918) even established a racial hierarchy of suitability for military service. In it, North Africans were considered particularly suited to acts of brutality and praised as first-line soldiers. However, Porot and Hesnard also noted the impulsivity of North Africans, which put them at risk for hysteria; therefore, they recommended that this population be supervised closely. Of all North Africans, psychiatrists of the time characterized only Muslims as posing particular problems; this conclusion was linked to Muslims' alleged resistance to civilized modernity, technological order, and military discipline.

Colonial psychiatry literature triggered an explosion of interest in primitivism in postwar France and contributed to French philosopher Lucien Lévy-Bruhl's (1923) famous work, *Primitive Mentality*. Rather than the biological, Lévy-Bruhl evoked cultural and environmental factors as causes of primitive mentality. According to his perspective, the minds of people deemed primitive could, through "psychological and psychiatric instruction," be reversed in "the fulfillment of France's civilizing mission" (Keller 2007, 133). The interest in primitive mentality in the interwar period also "indicated that an ethnological subspecialty was gaining steam within the French psychiatric profession" (Keller 2007, 136). Psychiatrists practicing in North Africa insisted that close contact with colonial patients revealed the practical and political importance of specific, rather than general, ethnopsychiatric knowledge. Their work departed significantly from that of their metropolitan colleagues; their insistence on the biological nature of psychological constitution was aimed at forging local, pro-colonial political advocacy.

With the independence movements in the 1950s, ethnopsychiatric knowledge gained traction within yet another group: the French army's newly founded Fifth Bureau, which led psychological operations during the Algerian war. Keller (2007) notes that in response to Algerian Front de Libération Nationale (FLN, National Liberation Front) propaganda, this French unit developed strategies to convince Algerians of the benefits of French presence. They used press censorship, loud-speaker announcements, and street flyers to influence public opinion, which they believed could only be accomplished if the psychological characteristics of the "normal" North African were taken into account.

In France, medical journals and scholars enthusiastically received the work by the Algiers School and praised it for advancing psychiatric knowledge through a wealth of clinical experience. However, some French psychiatrists voiced dissent— particularly those who worked with migrants in the metropole and who attributed the high prevalence of mental disorders to feelings of nostalgia and dislocation rather than to intrinsic fatalism, impulsivity, or general deviance as described by the Algiers School (Alliez and Descombes 1952). But with the outbreak of the Algerian war in 1954, there was an influx of migrant populations to France, and general fears of instability exacerbated scathing representations of migrants within the medical and public spheres. Media outlets linked North Africans' alleged "tribal ways" to higher crime rates, which drew the attention of police authorities and led to migrants being characterized as innately criminal, deviant, and unable to assimilate.[1]

Other Colonial Psychiatry Approaches in Sub-Saharan Africa

Not all French psychiatric practice of the colonial period relied on a biologically racist paradigm. Before independence movements, other analyses emerged that were more nuanced and sketched the beginnings of a critical perspective on the colonial enterprise. Among them, French ethnologist and psychiatrist Octave Mannoni's *Psychologie de la colonisation* (1949), later published in English as *Prospero and Caliban* (1950), was based in the French colony of Madagascar and offered the first psychological study to problematize the colonial relationship itself. Mannoni considered the colonial situation an encounter that created relations of dependence between two kinds of personality: an inferior one (the colonized) and a superior one (the colonizer). He noted how a "dependency complex" among the Malagasy prefigured the arrival of the Europeans and explained their uncon-scious compliance with colonization.

Mannoni's innovation was his attention to the psychology of the colo-nizer, which he considered dominated by the same "perverse and infantile needs" as colonial subjects (McCulloch 1995, 102). He believed that colonizers were illegitimate representatives of European civilization and were responsible for colonial racism. To Mannoni (1950), racism was an aberration. Reflecting on the Malagasy revolt against French colonizers in 1947—one of the bloodiest episodes of the colonial period in Africa—Mannoni argued from a psychoanalytical perspective that what the Malagasy sought "was not political rights but relief from fear of abandonment. They wanted to project their own shortcomings onto Europeans and so they behaved like impossible children who wanted one thing but demanded another. If they were granted self-government at the wrong time, they would simply regress" (McCulloch 1995, 103). His interpretation relied on the analysis of Malagasy dreams, in which the theme of terror was recurrent. The limit of such an interpretation, however, was that it depoliticized distress by approaching independence strictly as a psychological problem while ignoring the economic and political demands made by the Malagasy during riots.

Generally, throughout the accounts of colonial psychiatrists of the time, colonized societies were characterized as diseased, mentally backward, or prone to mental illness. Even on the eve of independence and at a time of various social transitions, many psychiatrists maintained that the colonized—Africans in particular—lacked the ability to change or adapt to modern, urban environments. Their critique was also directed at African intellectuals who led nationalist movements for independence. These intellectuals "were portrayed as having the worst possible qualities for political leadership, combining an inability to accept responsibility or to show initiative with a predisposition to mental illness" (McCulloch 1995, 120). In this way, colonial psychiatry accounts also attempted to curtail potential political insurgence.

During the history of colonial France, two generalizing, monolithic representations of North and sub-Saharan Africans were disseminated and naturalized through colonial psychiatry's literature. They stand almost in opposition to each another: North Africans were depicted as religious fanatics, cunning, violent, and naturally subject to committing crimes. Sub-Saharan Africans were infantilized and shown to be mentally and socially backward, as well as irresponsible (Comaroff 1985). Colonial psychiatry thus contributed to the production of a tacit knowledge that supports racist representations of the same populations in France today. These populations continue to be characterized in monolithic ways using the same binary oppositions: *les Arabes* (Arabs), *les musulmans* (Muslims), *les Africains* (Africans), or *les noirs* (blacks). Derogatory representations, such as the "fanatic Muslim" or the "lazy African," have weakened over time, as the notion of biological racism has become delegitimized, but they are intermittently resurrected in both political and everyday discourse (Ndiaye 2008).

Voices of Dissent: The Emerging Field of Ethnopsychiatry and Frantz Fanon's Critique

In the context of colonial independence movements, some psychiatrists, psychologists, and anthropologists sought to deconstruct colonial psychiatry's premise of the primitive mind. Dr. Louis Mars (1953), a Haitian psychiatrist passionate about voodoo practices and politically engaged in decolonization activities, was the first to coin the term "ethnopsychiatry." The word would later be used by Hungarian anthropologist and psychoanalyst Georges Devereux, during his seminar at the Ecole Pratique des Hautes Etudes in Paris. Like other "ethno" disciplines, ethnopsychiatry defends the idea that peoples with no written tradition developed other systems of knowledge. Ethnopsychiatry thus implies that there are cultural variations of what we call the science of psychiatry. Georges Devereux (1970) was the first to formulate a clinical approach based on the complementary use of anthropology and psychoanalysis. This approach thus rejected the ethnocentric views of colonial psychiatry.

At the time, however, it was psychiatrist Frantz Fanon who offered the most passionate critique of colonial psychiatry and the political foundations on which it rested. Fanon did not work directly within the field that came to be called "ethnopsychiatry," but his denunciation of the political and human abuses of colonial psychiatry and his theorizing around racism and the impact of the sociopolitical environment on individuals' mental health have nevertheless influenced the emerging discipline (Youssef and Fadl 1996).

Born and raised in Martinique, Fanon received his medical education and degree in psychiatry in France. During this time, he encountered many North African men who had migrated to France as part of the labor force. He found that public hospitals treated these men with the utmost contempt, particularly when they presented themselves with vague complaints that physicians dubbed "the North African Syndrome" (Fanon 1952). Often, patients would be sent home with treatments with which they failed to comply and would later return to the hospital with similar complaints. Hospital staff perceived them as "malingerers" who used their fictitious ailments to escape work. This perception persisted for decades and was known in France as *sinistrose*, the colloquial translation of "malingering." Of course, this representation characterized North African migrant workers in the public imagination as illegitimate residents. While *sinistrose* arguably pointed to illness resulting from structural conditions of expatriation and racism, it was not recognized as such within clinic spaces; recognition would entail admitting the relationship between suffering and the precarious social conditions endured by migrant workers.

After obtaining his degree, Fanon left for Algeria, where he served as head of department at the Blida-Joinville Psychiatric Hospital until 1957, when he was deported for participating in FLN activities. He moved to Tunisia and died shortly thereafter. At Blida, he observed the provision of care to Muslim patients, wrote a brief review of ethnopsychiatric literature from British and Francophone Africa, and addressed the problem of effective care for inmates of colonial asylums. What distinguished Fanon's work from that of his peers was his sensitivity to both the sociocultural origins of his patients and the historical and political situations in which they lived (McCulloch 1995). To fully decolonize psychiatry as it was currently practiced and create more humane conditions within the hospital system, Fanon argued that a program of "socio-therapy" had to be implemented (Tosquelles 2001). However, when he tried to do so, he ran into a series of difficulties that ultimately caused his program to fail.

In an essay written with psychiatrist Jacques Azoulay (1954), Fanon described these difficulties, including the methodological problems that language and cultural barriers raised for proper therapeutic work. He argued, too, that the practice of psychiatry was self-defeating in a colonial context. How could psychiatrists work toward freeing patients from their psychological distress when colonization alienated them from their own environments? What Fanon highlighted were the structural conditions that oppressed patients outside asylum walls. In *The Wretched of the Earth*, Fanon (1973) reflects on his experience at Blida and theorizes the psychological consequences of colonial rule and oppression. As Cameroonian philosopher Achille Mbembe (2013, 254) has noted, Fanon's work continues to resonate because colonialism provided the basis for global capitalism, a related context in which the contemporary oppressed can be found among those whose access to rights are denied—those deemed "illegal"—and whose very presence seems to threaten our own existence and well-being.

LABOR MIGRATION IN THE METROPOLE

Labor migration began in France as industrialization expanded during a period of economic growth in the nineteenth century. Initially, migration was internal and flowed from rural to urban areas. However, this proved insufficient to support the necessary workforce, and French officials instituted an open-door policy for foreign migrant workers. Hargreaves (1995) reports that the foreign population in France increased steadily until the economic slump of the 1930s. Growth rates again grew during the *trente glorieuses* (the three economically flourishing decades following World War II) but have stabilized at around 6 percent since the mid-1970s (Hargreaves 1995). Until the 1960s, most laborers came from neighboring European countries. After that, workers increasingly came from Turkey, North Africa (particularly Algeria), and West Africa (primarily the Sahel region, including Mali, Mauritania, and Senegal).

French historian and political scientist Patrick Weil (2008) argues that France first elaborated a politics of immigration between the two world wars. State officials called on population experts to elaborate laws that would regulate the influx of immigrants and redefine access to French citizenship. Weil notes that experts' reports were often tainted by models of racial differentiation and hierarchy that circulated widely at the time and were concerned with establishing "degrees of possible assimilation" (2008, 24–26). The resulting immigration politics ranked workers according to their nationality, physical appearance, regularity, production, discipline, and understanding of the French language. "Arabs" were ranked at the bottom of the scale and characterized as fatalist and gullible; Jews were also identified as racially undesirable (Weil 2008, 33–34). Population experts during this period encouraged a national immigration policy based on "ethnic quality" (Weil 2008, 54).

In the aftermath of World War II, labor migration was encouraged to compensate for the country's weak demographic growth, but "successive governments sought as far as possible to encourage European rather than African or Asian immigrants" (Hargreaves 1995, 11). Despite this, labor migration originating in the Maghreb (Algeria, Morocco, Tunisia) grew rapidly. Unlike most European migrants who settled in France with their families, most North African workers arrived alone, returned to their countries of origin after a few years, and were replaced by others in their village on a rotating basis (Sayad 2004). These migrant workers were concentrated in the centers of industrial urban areas as early as the Second French Empire (1852–1870) (Noiriel 1988). In 1956, the Société nationale de construction de logement pour les travailleurs algériens (SONACOTRA, National Society for the Construction of Housing for Algerian Workers) was created to solve issues of unhealthy housing conditions. Male workers stayed in hostels (*foyers*), but employers encouraged the formation of ghettos to house families. According to French historian Gérard Noiriel, "Regrouping on an 'ethnic' basis by neighborhood or zone is a strategy explicitly defined by the employer seeking to reinforce the homogeneity and stability of the workforce" (1988, 172).

The assimilationist strategy of political officials, who sought to avoid the dangers of such ghettoization, was thus defeated by economic interests, which resulted in the exact opposite. With the urban renovation plan of the 1960s, migrant families were pushed into low-income housing projects in the suburbs, and priority urban zones emerged. In 1958, the government created a Fund for Social Action for Muslim Algerian workers. In 1966, it also created the Department of Population and Migrations as an umbrella ministry to encompass the former Departments of Work, Public Health, and Population. On July 3, 1974, labor immigration was suspended (except for members of the European Union). From then on, France unsuccessfully launched a series of various "voluntary return" programs, in which migrants were offered economic incentives to return to their home countries.

Separate Care for Foreigners: The Creation of the Avicenne Hospital

Between the world wars, France had the fastest-growing migrant population in the world. French authorities were fearful of the threats they imagined these migrants posed, particularly political unrest and crime, and were especially weary of North African colonial subjects. By 1930, as many as 100,000 North African workers had crossed the Mediterranean, entered France, and settled in the north-eastern outskirts of Paris. Many lived in small crowded rentals or hostels, and most were employed as low-skill laborers in the metallurgical and mining indus-tries, where they occupied the most physically strenuous positions. Only a few migrants entered as skilled workers, professionals, or students. Partly due to unsanitary living conditions, work hazards, and exposure to metallurgical chem-icals, there was a high prevalence of disease among these migrants. Scientific reports filled national newspapers, blaming migrants for bringing disease to the country but failing to acknowledge that "most of the immigrants in local hospi-tals had contracted their diseases, notably tuberculosis and syphilis, after they arrived in France. If foreigners were more likely to suffer from tuberculosis, as was generally believed, it had far more to do with the conditions in France than in their homelands" (Rosenberg 2006, 176).

Around this time, a French doctor practicing in Algeria, Professor Amédée Laffont, suggested the creation of a Parisian hospital adapted to the needs of Mus-lim patients from North Africa.[2] It was in this context that the government's deci-sion to build a hospital far from the city center was made: North African migrants not only constituted a political threat but also a public health risk in the eyes of officials. In building Avicenne, the administration actively tried to re-create a famil-iar environment for North African patients and adapt to the needs of this popu-lation. For example, Arabic- and Kabyle-speaking staff members were recruited or trained. Hospital nurses took language classes and were also taught the history and geography of North Africa. Even a prayer room and accommodations for dietary restrictions were established for Muslim patients and staff. However, Avicenne had its problems. The hiring of staff was questionable; the hospital attracted uncertified Muslim medical students from the Maghreb and largely overlooked public health standards. Even worse, it was located in an isolated area of a working-class suburb, next to a waste-treatment plant and away from public transportation. Rosenberg notes that most Muslim patients avoided the hospi-tal, which made them feel segregated from the rest of the population.

More than demonstrating governmental respect for difference, the building of a separate hospital fit with the biological racism of the time. In his study of immi-gration control in interwar Paris, American historian Clifford Rosenberg (2004) demonstrates that though the project to build such a hospital was underpinned by medical concerns about responding to the particular needs of foreign patients, it also reflected political concern around controlling colonized populations. Pierre Godin, then head of the North African brigade unit, argued that the hospital would "cleanse" (*blanchir*) foreigners (Rosenberg 2004, 652). Rosenberg documents how the Avicenne Hospital, once built, was linked to the Service de Surveillance et de Protection des Indigènes Nord-Africains (SSPINA, Surveillance and Protection

Services for North African Indigenous People). The relationship between caring for and regulating North African populations was thus articulated as clearly in the *métropole* (mainland France), as in the colonies.

The Illness of Immigration

In his analysis of French discourse on North African migrant workers, French sociologist Abdelmalek Sayad articulates how public representations of migrants affected their very relationships with their own bodies: "The body as representation and presentation of the self, the body as the seat of affect and of the intellect (for the body is inhabited by the entire group that lives inside us), the body as an instrument of labor and as site and expression of illness" (2004, 179). Illness, according to Sayad, provides the best insight into the contradictions that constitute the migrant condition: "Because the immigrant has no meaning, in either his own eyes or those of others, and because, ultimately, he has no existence except through his work, illness, perhaps even more so than the idleness it brings, is inevitably experienced as the negation of the immigrant" (2004, 180). Such contradictions initially stem from the fact that the conditions originally generating *emigration*, which produced the living conditions North African immigrants faced in France, were largely ignored in the popular discourse on migrants.[3] Instead, public discourse always focused on the "problems" migrants caused for French institutions.

Discursive references to "immigrants' problems," rather than France's problem with migrants, highlight the importance of naming and labeling practices in public discourse and their practical impact on the health of migrants and the management of migrants' health by institutional actors. For example, according to Sayad (2004, 179), public discourse on immigration deliberately overlooks the genesis of migrants' "problems" both to regulate a phenomenon that threatens the public order and to avoid questioning "what an immigrant is and what immigration is." Sayad (2004) notes that this paradox results from immigrants' illnesses being bound to their migrant condition: the more an immigrant struggles to recover his health, and therefore his life equilibrium, the more he tends to expect from medicine. Meanwhile, he points out, the medical establishment is willing to make some concessions for foreign patients, such as resorting to interpreters in hospitals, but its representatives refuse to take into account the social circumstances that generate migrants' illnesses and instead simply create an index of pathology (Sayad 2004)—as illustrated by the epidemic of *sinistrose*, mentioned earlier.

As foreigners, postwar labor migrants have therefore experienced ubiquitous suspicion (Bennani [1980] 2015) and surveillance in France over time. As a result, negative popular discourse around migrants, with roots in earlier colonial representations, continues to proliferate in the present.

CONFRONTING NEW POLITICS: EVOLVING
REPRESENTATIONS OF THE "MIGRANT" AND
THE EMERGENCE OF THE MENTAL HEALTH FIELD

In the 1960s, French psychiatry went through profound reform, sparked by the demise of the asylum system of mental health care. What took its place was a new system of district-based, outpatient psychiatric care, referred to as *sectorisation* (Petitjean and Leguay 2002). This period of reform also created space for the genesis of new clinical initiatives, such as voluntary mental health associations.[4] Early associations during this time focused on helping asylum seekers and interrogating the psychopathology of trauma. Examples include Centre Minkowska (then known as the Tiomkine dispensary), established in 1951, and the Center for Medical Advice to Asylum Seekers, created in 1979. Although these clinics' approaches to trauma varied, they were built on related universalist ideas: humans share a common psychic world and therefore a universalist experience of trauma, but expressions of symptoms and representations of suffering vary culturally (Fassin and Rechtman 2009).

The initial focus in this period was on postwar refugees and political asylum seekers. This is explained in part by the favorable legal status accorded to refugees at the Geneva Convention in 1951 and in the French Law of July 25, 1952, which led to the creation of the French Office for the Protection of Refugees and Stateless Persons (OFPRA). Human rights discourse of the time shaped the universalist clinical approach to mental health care for refugees. In the context of the Cold War, OFPRA called for tolerance and flexibility in the interpretation of criteria for obtaining refugee status. For a few decades, individuals were not required to present proof of political persecution or even hide their economic interest: the French government seemed to accept fleeing from communism as a self-evident collective motivation for immigration. From the 1950s to the 1970s, France welcomed Russians, Hungarians, Polish, Armenians, and Czechoslovakians (Akoka 2017, 56).

At the end of the 1970s, however, this favorable and compassionate view toward refugees changed. In the context of economic crisis, weakening welfare policies, and restrictions on labor migration, a climate of renewed suspicion about refugees' motives emerged. Procedures to obtain refugee status took longer and were the object of increasing administrative scrutiny. Around this time, the "asylum seeker" was born in political rhetoric and became a new administrative category. It corresponded to the transitory, liminal status foreigners experienced while their refugee applications were being examined (d'Halluin 2009). Popular distinctions were also made between refugees and economic migrants. People who continued to seek work became "bad economic migrants," while those who had chosen to remain in France and bring over their families were stigmatized as profiteers of the generous French welfare system.

From Workers to Families

Migration dynamics shifted significantly with legislation in 1976 that regulated family reunification (Barou 2002; La Documentation Française 2006). This legislation articulated the conditions under which male immigrants residing in France could legally bring spouses, children, and other relatives into the country. Family reunification policies attempted to mitigate the separation of labor migrants from their families, which was caused by the suspension of labor migration in 1974; this limited the possibility of circulatory migration between France and African countries.

Since the early 1980s, the resulting influx of foreign families has translated into negative stereotyping, discrimination, and feelings of threat to French national identity. While some scholars argue that North Africans are more vulnerable to racism and discrimination in contemporary France (Lamont 2000), I argue that sub-Saharan Africans have been the priority target of public health initiatives designed to manage "culturally different" migrant families. This is explained partly by the fact that political authorities have recently characterized sub-Saharan Africans as epitomizing illegal migration. The settling of African households in Paris and its suburbs "generated public awareness of large families living in inadequate lodgings. . . . In conjunction with the pronatalist family allocation system, the perceived costs to the state of high fertility among sub-Saharan African women emerged as an increasingly controversial public issue" (Sargent 2005, 148). Beyond economics, this presence of large families was used by France's most vocal anti-immigration party, the National Front, to target polygamy and Islam as moral threats to the nation. Polygamy was implicitly tolerated by the French government until the passage of the Pasqua Laws in 1993, which threatened all men who remained in polygamous unions and their wives—with the exception of the first wife—with the loss of their residence and work permits and subsequent deportation.

Many women who moved to France to join their husbands had little formal education, urban experience, or French language skills (Nicollet 1992). For them, social workers and biomedical practitioners served as front-line and principle sources of initiation into everyday life. They came with concerns about housing, documentation, employment, child-rearing, the educational system, and marital disputes. These dilemmas fell under the purview of numerous state institutions—schools, hospitals, local government, and the criminal justice system, to name a few—and were challenging to manage. State agents perceived dilemmas as cultural in origin or the result of language barriers and frequently resorted to community interpreters and subsequently to "cultural mediators" to communicate with non-French-speaking migrants. These efforts were often directed at women, who frequently interacted with state institutions in the context of maternal and child health care (Charte MCS 2006; Quiminal and Timera 2002). Cultural mediation thus emerged as a formal profession in this era of exploratory approaches to public health interventions with migrants.

During the 1990s, migrants and their families continued to be characterized as living "off the largesse of welfare payments" (Wieviorka 2002). The government pursued the restriction of migration flows and moved toward a policy of "zero immigration" (Viet 1998). A series of laws and amendments addressing gender, marital status, and family composition thus successively threatened African migrants (Sargent 2005). More recently, entire immigrant families—including French raised and educated children—were targeted for deportation (*Le Monde* 2005). Such restrictive policies have increased the number of undocumented migrants, leading to increased economic precarity within migrant populations.

Simultaneously, France has promoted a republican model of migrant integration based on a logic of universal rights, which categorically denies the relevance of ethnic differences. But the November 2005 migrant riots clearly demonstrated the failure of this long-standing state model of integration, occurring as they did amid widespread protests of discrimination among immigrant populations (Tshimanga, Gondola, and Bloom 2009). The government's response to this crisis was emblematic of a profound philosophical contradiction: despite the collective protest of social inequalities, state officials depicted the uprising as the product of unassimilated migrant families breeding delinquent and psychologically distressed youth (Le Goaziou and Muchielli 2006).

In contemporary France, migrants—especially those of North and sub-Saharan African origin—are perceived as a marked threat to the social order. Certain cultural practices have been identified as particularly problematic. For example, the minister of employment denounced polygamy as a possible cause of urban violence (*Le Monde* 2005), and the minister of the interior proposed a medical plan to treat the "psychological and psychiatric disorders" causing delinquency among "migrants' children" (Ministère de l'Interieur 2005). The term "delinquency of exclusion" was coined, linking "the foreign or immigrant delinquent to inherited cultural pathologies and dangerous social milieus" (Terrio 2009, 13). Meanwhile, media coverage of youth crime in the *banlieues* (suburbs) popularly associated migrants with insecurity, which had constituted a major political issue during past presidential elections.

CHANGING REPRESENTATIONS OF MIGRANT FAMILIES AND THE BROADENING OF THE MENTAL HEALTH FIELD

During the 1980s, France experienced a period of economic recession, characterized by long-term unemployment and violence in what became known as "sensitive neighborhoods" (*quartiers en difficulté*).[5] New language in political discourse was then created to interpret these new forms of poverty and urban violence.

Social policies took the form of stipends for the unemployed and youth programs to prevent delinquency and facilitate social integration.[6]

Thus, what became known as "the social issue" (*la question sociale*) in public discourse shaped politics throughout the 1990s. This phenomenon was formally coined "social exclusion" in a series of government-mandated reports.[7] This state-defined notion, albeit ambiguous, signaled a change in perspective about the nation's poor and excluded. While they were considered maladapted and delinquent before the 1970s (Fassin 2004), this new rhetoric around exclusion, with its accompanying social policies, characterized both categories as *victims* who *suffered* from social inequalities. As a result, the term "suffering" gained social valence as a category subsuming a wide array of social problems, including "the suffering of the unemployed, the suffering of drug users, the students suffering from failing at school, the immigrants suffering from exile, [and] foreign-born youth suffering from discrimination" (Fassin 2004, 26).

This new discourse on suffering highlighted not social inequalities but individual experience. One way this understanding of suffering became legitimized was through the institutionalization of counseling: a form of professional therapeutic listening that engaged a wide array of state actors, particularly in the public and mental health sectors. This new form of therapeutic listening—situated somewhere between social services and psychiatry—functionally extended the boundaries of mental health outside traditional psychiatry and psychology services in the country. Fassin (2004) argues that the institutionalization of therapeutic listening resulted as much from a concern with caring for the excluded as with regulating them.

Together, I suggest, these events produced a "universe of possibilities" (Bourdieu 1991, 10) for a new form of ethnopsychiatry to emerge on the French public health landscape. Indeed, this discursive shift to notions of migrants as suffering individual victims—and the rise of counseling to address their suffering—to some extent fit in with older pathologizing notions in the history of French ethnopsychiatry, all of which (past and present) cast cultural difference as pathological.

Tobie Nathan's School of Ethnopsychiatry

The first ethnopsychiatry clinic was launched in France in 1980 by charismatic psychologist Tobie Nathan. Nathan opened his practice at the aforementioned Avicenne Hospital in Bobigny, a northern suburb of Paris. At the time, this location was symbolically charged as the first specialized health institution serving the needs of Muslim patients from North Africa, and its administration struggled to do this well. The hospital's head of child and adolescent psychiatry, Professor Serge Lebovici, invited Nathan to help him better serve the needs of migrant populations, and they formed an alliance to create the first ethnopsychiatry consultation in France.

Although greatly inspired by the teachings of his mentor, Georges Devereux, Nathan's clinical practice significantly deviated from Devereux's own theoretical clinical complementarity model.[8] In Devereux's model, he contends that anthropology and psychiatry should play complementary roles in the treatment of psychopathology. In contrast, while Nathan framed the intellectual genealogy of his clinic in relation to Devereux's model, he did not elicit the input or participation of anthropologists.

Rather, Nathan constituted a body of experts, called "ethno-clinical mediators," whose competence was evaluated based on their belonging to a patient's ethnic group or on their knowledge of one or several languages of a cultural area. These mediators played the role of ethnologist's informant for Nathan (Andoche 2001). In doing so, Nathan broke away from the careful distinction in Devereux's model between a universal expression of "culture in itself" and local expressions of culture. Instead, he substituted the concept of culture as a closed, all-determining system in the expression of mental disorders (Nathan 1986). In Nathan's model, the psyche is subordinated to culture. His theory, called "cultural closure," postulates that migrant patients can only be treated in their cultural system and in reference to "traditional" typologies (Mestre 2006, 168–169). This conclusion led Nathan to devise a method of therapeutic practice that was an adaptation of African village assemblies and that he considered akin to "African" healing. In this model, ethno-clinical mediators joined patients in a session and circulated discourse in a particular manner: each ethno-clinician (also called co-therapist) spoke in turn to the issues presented by the patient. This co-therapy team sometimes also used ritual objects in therapy or other rituals, such as divination (Andoche 2001).

Pushing Cultural Relativism, Loosening Institutional Legitimacy

A decade later, in 1993, Nathan created the Georges Devereux Center as another consultation service, housed in the psychology department of the University of Paris 8, where ethnopsychiatry as a discipline was provided space to experiment with the concept of mediation. Patients were referred to the Devereux Center through second intention by another medical, social, education, or justice institution.[9] The center therefore operated through "in network" (*en réseau*) referrals from state institutions, to which it also offered diagnostic and therapeutic advice, workshops on working with immigrant families, training or information on ethnopsychiatry, and cultural expertise. Nathan's clinic built its institutional authority by becoming a site for therapy, research, and teaching, while simultaneously intersecting with state agents across institutional boundaries. The George Devereux Center conducted as many as six hundred consultations a year, not counting outside interventions within social services, health-promoting associations, and justice tribunals (Fassin 2000). Colleagues and students of Nathan, who reflected on the popularity of his center, often commented in public meetings that

Nathan was worshipped like a guru and even had the spellbinding aura of a sorcerer; indeed, he used his charisma to conduct rituals during consultations (Andoche 2001).

In 1994, amid a changing climate of increasingly conservative, anti-immigration discourse, Nathan attempted to extend his authority and establish scientific legitimacy for the French practice of ethnopsychiatry by publishing *L'influence qui guérit* (A healing influence). Around this time, a republican model of migrant integration, based on a logic of universal rights that denies the relevance of ethnic differences, had gained favor within the government, and certain cultural practices had become punishable by law.[10] In the media, ethnic difference was being characterized in denigrating terms.[11] The philosophy of Nathan's book marked a definitive rupture with the culturalist political ideology, which allowed his initial meteoric rise in public opinion. Under the weight of this changing tide of public opinion about migrants, Nathan's book denounced common psychiatric methods used with migrant patients as ineffective and presented a virulent assault on Western psychiatry.

Nathan rejected Western psychoanalytical theory's notion of psychic universality, retaining only the Western understanding of influence as a technique by which patients' mental health states could be modified. "In other words," he noted, "I am not far from thinking that psychology—as a science of the psychic apparatus, following Freud's formula, . . . would be a pure fiction. The only defendable scientific discipline would be, forgive the barbarism, an influence-ology, which object would be to analyze the different procedures to modify the other" (1994, 21). More broadly, Nathan used the book to critically analyze modern medicine's claim to rationality and legitimacy via its reference to the theoretico-experimental model of modern science (Stengers and Nathan 1995). In doing so, Nathan not only confronted the medical establishment but tried to illustrate how medicine reinforced specific political ideology that caused actual suffering for migrants.

Nathan began a political struggle against what he called "the constraint of humanity" (1994, 143) and showed how migrants in France suffered from an institutional rejection of their cultural difference and from being forced to assimilate as "universal" beings. Such assimilation policies, he argued, were directly detrimental to immigrants' well-being. He even attributed the abnormal number of infantile cases of autism he encountered among migrants' children to national assimilation policies; he located their cause within the experience of immigration and a family's loss of its cultural environment. Further, he suggested that France's assimilation policies and its "machines of cultural abrasion" (e.g., clinics and schools) (1994, 191) damaged the very psychological structure of migrant individuals. While Nathan's problematization of the higher incidence of mental health disorders among migrants and their children was justified, the vehemence and extreme cultural relativistic nature of his accusations ultimately undermined his legitimacy, the cogence of his theory, and the richness of his clinical experience.

Following the publication of *L'influence qui guérit*, critiques of Nathan abounded. The delegitimization of his work and reputation occurred through the circulation of scientific critiques in journals (Dahoun 1992; Douville and Ottavi 1995; Fassin 1999) and through lay discourse in newspapers and magazines (Benslama 1996; Policar 1997; Sibony 1997). Both social scientists and psychiatrists disparaged Nathan's cultural relativistic stance and his pathologization of the political through willful misrecognition of the structural violence that affected migrants. For example, Fassin (2000) noted that for Nathan, migrants are Bambara or Fulani individuals first and foremost and must be treated as such. They are never understood as migrants facing visa difficulties, encountering housing discrimination, or confronting everyday racism in France. "Difference so construed," Fassin argued, "can only lead to a construction of difference void of any social substance, and to a reassuring sublimation of conflict, which is the principle of politics" (2000, 19). Psychiatrists in particular denounced Nathan's deconstruction and reappropriation of psychoanalysis. Richard Rechtman, a French psychiatrist and anthropologist conducting research on psychiatric disorders among Cambodian refugees, argued that Nathan's work was based on "abusive simplifications of ethnopsychoanalysis" (1995, 120). Further, Rechtman noted the racial undertones of Nathan's extreme relativism and said that by "suggesting the existence of fundamental differences between the functioning of the human psyche according to one individual's culture of origin risks not only to reactivate the concept of race, which paradoxically he claims to actively contest in his militancy, but also to inaugurate a theory of human species based on ethnic belonging" (1995, 125). From that point, Nathan was publicly cast as a heretic, refusing to circumscribe his speech to medical orthodoxy or to the rules of French republican universalism.

From my perspective, Nathan's discourse was intended to recontextualize what medical and republican ideologies had sought to decontextualize through sponsoring ethnopsychiatry: the relevance of culturally sensitive care in improving mental health provision for migrants and in unveiling unhealthy consequences of the structural conditions of immigration and of the French "integration" model. Notably, Nathan's approach was received differently in Italy, where clinicians mainly retained his innovative work on the symbolic meaning of traditional healing practices and their possible articulations with psychotherapy but set aside his provocative remarks (Giordano 2014). Nathan's supporters in France—anthropologist Bruno Latour and Belgian philosopher Isabelle Stengers (1997)—have written about how Nathan's work suffered from the backlash caused by a specific ideological framework in which discussion about culture was always embedded between ethnic or group (*communautariste*) definitions and references to the republic and citizenship. As a result, Nathan's ethnopsychiatry was discursively characterized as an irrational science, or even charlatanism and sorcery, and thus opposed to republican-friendly universal science.

TRANSCULTURAL PSYCHIATRY, TRAUMA, AND CONTEMPORARY FIGURES OF "MIGRANT SUFFERING"

Following the public critique of Nathan's school of ethnopsychiatry, all special-ized mental health institutions in France were forced to adapt their theoretical premises. Centre Minkowska—established long before Nathan's ethnopsychiatry initiative and discussed in chapter 2—adapted easily. For other institutions, this was not the case. Clinicians at Avicenne Hospital, who were trained by Nathan, now acknowledge the negative implications of Nathan's culturally essentialist posi-tion (Moro, de La Noë, and Mouchenick 2006). But while they recognize that a separate, specialized model of mental health-care provision for immigrants may stigmatize such patients, they argue that it is necessary in the current French health-care context. As the director of one center noted, in an ideal public health system, specialized care would be unnecessary.[12] Theoretically, the recent special-ized health-care model acknowledges social precarity as a core factor of psycho-logical distress among many migrants and partly inscribes itself within the movement of psychosocial medicine.

These institutions continue to underscore the importance of cultural exper-tise (Sargent and Larchanché 2009), and they use discourse that strives to uphold French public health ideology promoting healthcare access for all while seeking medical and social science sanctioning (Larchanché 2010). Indeed, I argue that the discourse of French republicanism, clothed in the language of science, imposes a "sphere of communicability" that is "crucial for boundary work, for the creation and maintenance of boundaries, and for the regulation of membership" (Briggs 2005, 274). In France, republicanism is the official state discourse—a set of nor-mative institutional ideologies and practices—"against which all linguistic prac-tices are objectively measured" and gain legitimacy (Bourdieu 1991, 44). The survival of specialized mental health centers thus partly relied on their capacity to adhere to the limits of what Bourdieu called this "unified linguistic market" (1991, 45). I do not, however, ignore the conceptual transformations that had to take place for this change of paradigm.

Currently, person-centered transcultural psychiatry provides a rallying approach that builds on the cultural competence approach (Kirmayer 2012) along with its critiques (Metzl and Hansen 2014). In other words, transcultural psychi-atry has integrated contemporary, dynamic definitions of culture and its relation to psychological distress, and has critically addressed the impact of stigma and inequality within mental health delivery on the production of distress itself. In France, most transcultural psychiatry consultations are concentrated in Paris. A well-known one is the Avicenne consultation, led until recently by child psy-chiatrist Marie Rose Moro, the most prominent figure in transcultural psychiatry in France, and Centre Minkowska. However, the increasing number of clini-cians trained in the transcultural psychiatry approach has gradually led to the creation of transcultural consultations in other major French cities, most of which are organized as associations, operating with more limited means and more or less legitimacy.

Contemporary Migrations

Demographer and anthropologist François Héran (2017) has established that since 2002, the number of residence permits issued to extra-European migrants in France has remained stable. Among the average 200,000 permits delivered each year, most are awarded to spouses of French citizens, to international students, or for family reunification. On average, only 10 percent are awarded to asylum seekers, which minimizes France's self-image as a generous land of refuge. In 2014, when the European Union received 122,000 asylum requests (much less than Turkey, Greece, Jordan, or Lebanon), Germany awarded asylum protection to 26,000 Syrians, Switzerland to 17,000, France to 2,000, and Great Britain to 1,500 (Héran in *L'Express* 2015).

Regardless, restrictive immigration and asylum policies have not stopped migrants from coming. Increasingly, those who survive the journey often arrive in a state of great psychological distress or trauma. Illegal arrivals in Europe have been stable since the 1980s, but their importance and character changed dramatically during 2014, following violence in the Middle East as the Islamic State consolidated its position in Iraq and Syria. A wave of factors has motivated such illegal entries: armed intervention in Libya in 2011, civil war in Syria the same year, ethnic war in South Sudan in 2013, continuing civil war in Afghanistan, and instability in the Balkans. Sea crossing via the Mediterranean has become a major immigration route; departure points have been defined by various conflicts in Syria, Libya, Iraq, and East Africa (particularly Sudan, Eritrea, and Somalia) and linked to greater border control in transit countries, such as Morocco, or destination points, such as Spain. According to the International Organization for Migration, the numbers of deaths while crossing the Mediterranean skyrocketed during 2011, 2014, and 2015 (Fargues 2016, 2–3).

A generalized pattern is that people are increasingly prevented from achieving legal immigration and becoming "integrated": they become stuck in a liminal state of migration, bearing the stigma of social pariah (Agier 2017, 23). One example is the Dublin agreement (last ratified in 2014), which by trying to regulate and thus reduce asylum requests in Europe have in fact produced delays and irregularities in asylum procedures that have prejudiced asylum seekers and worsened the precarity of their situations. Through this system, many are forced to apply for asylum in the country of first entry, such as Italy or Greece, when the majority actually seek residence in countries like France or the United Kingdom. As a result, those who refuse to stay in their country of entry continue their journey but find themselves in a state of administrative limbo; they cannot reapply for asylum within the two years following the filing of their first application, which often occurs without their consent at the same time their fingerprints are taken by authorities. Among increasingly vehement opposition between members of the European Union regarding immigration regulations, countries of first entry have recently refused the responsibility of fingerprinting incoming immigrants, thus declining their country's responsibility for processing all asylum requests. People who find themselves in this liminal state are so numerous, they have come to constitute a new social category: the "dublined."

Another social category arising from recent immigration patterns is the "unaccompanied minor" (*mineurs non accompagnés*)—a term that evolved from another French term, "isolated foreign minors" (*mineurs isolés étrangers*). The phenomenon of unaccompanied minor migrants was first noted in the early 2000s and has increased ever since. Until the creation in 2013 of a special unit for the protection, evaluation, and orientation of unaccompanied minors (Dispositif national de mise à l'abri, d'évaluation et d'orientation des jeunes mineurs isolés étrangers), there were no reliable data on their numbers. Recent figures indicate that they increased from 5,990 in 2015 to 8,054 in 2016 (Ministère de la Justice 2017, 5). Seventy-one percent of these minor migrants come from the African continent (44 percent from West Africa, 27 percent from the Sahel) (Ministère de la Justice 2016, 7). Although this type of immigration remains low, it has attracted much attention from all segments of society. As children, these migrants often arouse compassion. However, their youth does not protect them from the strong climate of suspicion that currently shrouds all types of immigration (Bricaud 2006). The media has often used them for sensational news by documenting their petty delinquency (pickpocketing) or addressing situations of their exploitation (prostitution networks, illegal work in sweatshops). A recent study offers a typology of these unaccompanied minors around four archetypal figures: the exiled, the mandated, the aspiring, and the exploited (Etiemble and Zanna 2013). Young migrants often find themselves at the crossroads of two types of public intervention: those aiming at regulating immigration and those relying on child protection policies. Among the second, unaccompanied minors have been the object of interest and clinical propositions for transcultural psychiatry clinicians (among them Benoit de Coignat and Baubet 2013; Mahyeux, 2017; Radjack, Guzman, and Moro 2014).

Trauma and Social Precarity

The violence of contemporary migration journeys, as well as the stark conditions in camps, transit zones, and destination countries alike, predispose individuals to psychological distress at best and trauma at worst. Such conditions have contributed to the popularization of a "clinic of trauma" (Capogna-Bardet 2014), a clinical approach specifically dedicated to trauma survivors and in which transcultural psychiatry occupies an influential position. The post-traumatic stress disorder (PTSD) diagnosis has become pivotal within health-care delivery to migrants, asylum seekers, and refugees (d'Halluin 2009; Sturm, Baubet, and Moro 2010). Scientific literature points to a high prevalence of this diagnosis among migrants (d'Halluin 2009; Kirmayer et al. 2010; Sturm, Baubet, and Moro 2010), and some scholars suggest that all "forced" migrants display PTSD symptoms to some extent (Copping, Shakespeare-Finch, and Paton 2010). What the literature also indicates is the risk for this diagnostic construction to downplay or even ignore cultural, linguistic, or sociopolitical contexts and determinants of health. However, these factors often deeply influence experiences interpreted as traumatic, their symptomatic manifestation, and distress and recovery narratives (Beneducce 2016; Fassin and d'Halluin 2005; Fassin and Rechtman 2009; Goguikian Ratcliff 2012; Kirmayer et al. 2010; Young 1995). This same body of scholarship has established the limits of PTSD as a diagnosis for migrants: it individualizes and pathologizes trauma, focuses narrowly on premigration events, and thus denies the existence of trauma experienced during and after migration, such as social precarity and uncertainty about the future.

Overall, the contours of the social representation of migrants seem to have gradually moved from a focus on the cultural "other" to a concern with their precarity. The figure of the "precarious migrant" has emerged as a new "overwhelming figure" (Chambon 2013) challenging the training and competence of professionals. The emergence of clinical paradigms other than transcultural psychiatry, such as the clinical approach to exile (Benslama 2004) or the clinical approach to trauma (Baubet et al. 2004), seems to indicate a need for new clinical and therapeutic modes of intervention. Transcultural psychiatry has been a strong advocate of caring practices that are sensitive to individuals' structural vulnerability. This has translated into ways of organizing clinics that promote partnership with local actors involved in assisting migrants in various realms (legal paperwork, housing, social services, schooling). Of the new approaches that have emerged, transcultural psychiatry professionals are most vocal in denouncing contemporary social and cultural health inequalities. In that respect, they constitute major advocates for the mandatory use of interpreter services in all public health institutions, as well as for the training of all professionals who assist migrants.

Some scholars, such as Didier Fassin (2006), have been critical of the primacy of the "social issue" in French psychiatry and psychology discourse. They denounce counseling as a new form of governance through listening, which masks inequalities and reifies exclusion and suffering through a register of compassion. Fassin wonders "why, in societies hostile to immigrants and lacking in concern for undesirable others, there remains a sense of common humanity collectively expressed through attention to human needs and suffering" (2006, 366). In the remainder of this book, I show that transcultural psychiatry professionals, namely those working at Centre Minkowska, are well aware of this paradox and regularly wrestle with the risks of pathologizing situations that relate to state agents' inability to find support outlets for their migrant clients who face conditions of extreme precarity. The work of identifying which part of the problem rests within social hardships and which within psychological distress is difficult, to say the least, as both are so often intertwined. In the everyday reality of the clinic, in which staff members use logics of caregiving to decide what counts as a legitimate referral to a specialized mental health clinic, we will see that what is theoretically easy to denounce becomes ethically more complex and challenging.

*   *   *

The successive understandings, representations, and characterizations of migrants and their problems, along with the specific clinical initiatives they have inspired, have thus evolved in close relation to the political context in which they emerged. While I believe it is helpful to understand how the political subjectification of migrants partly informed the regulative basis of specialized institutional interventions, we must not lose sight of the many practical challenges that also arise in the institutional management of migrants: language barriers, conflicting representations of health and disease, and disagreements on the course of treatment. (For a poignant illustration of such issues, see Fadiman 1997.) These challenges, if unacknowledged, may negatively affect the caring foundations of both social and health services to migrants.

The tension I articulate throughout this book, between caring and regulating, is not intended to blame any specific institutional effort to address migrants. The macro-analysis I have adopted for this genealogy of migrant suffering, combined with the scholarship I have relied on to shape my argument, may indicate the opposite; but my goal is to call attention to the complexity of the dilemmas raised in the everyday management of migrant patients and their recent referrals to specialized mental health centers. The ethnography that follows is intended to bring this nuance to the fore.

2 · TRANSCULTURAL PRACTICE AT CENTRE MINKOWSKA

Centre Minkowska has seven consultation offices lining both sides of a long hallway, which ends with the director's office and a large room used for teaching, seminars, and staff meetings. Other than the consultation offices, which are numbered and assigned to therapists, rooms are given a name. My office is named after the leader of the Palo Alto group, American anthropologist and psychologist Gregory Bateson, who helped develop the systemic approach to psychiatry and introduced the concept of the "double bind" within research on schizophrenia.[1] The coffee room is named after Vincent van Gogh—a passionate research subject for Françoise Minkowska, who published a book concluding that the famous artist suffered not from schizophrenia but from glischroid epilepsy. A reproduction of one of Van Gogh's famous self-portraits, painted by a now-retired secretary, hangs on one of the coffee room's walls. The meeting room farther down the hall is named after psychiatrist Jean-Pierre M'Barga, who led the African consultation during the center's early days and has since passed away. Another meeting room is named after American anthropologist Margaret Mead, a famous figure of the culture and personality school of thought. The names of these rooms reflect the contemporary culture of Centre Minkowska as an institution. The center supports interdisciplinarity through collaborations between anthropology and psychology and approaches that focus on a combination of the universal and the specific. It also illustrates Dr. Rachid Bennegadi's influence in shaping Centre Minkowska's contemporary clinical approach.

The center has a strong institutional identity. Stories about its epistemological evolution circulate regularly among the staff during coffee breaks or even formal meetings. Everyone who visits or works here is briefed about its past. As I show later, this desire to constantly narrate the center's history relates to staff members' need to make sense of its present relevance—particularly in a context where it is often narrowly characterized by others as a source of cultural expertise and a specialized center in charge of caring for foreigners. In response, staff members debate the center's position within contemporary public health theory and practice, and reassert the general importance of its contemporary person-centered approach. This constant narration around the role of the center acts as an expression of collective ethos as people try to make sense of the contradictions inherent in specialized mental health provision in France.

In this chapter, I highlight the ethics of the center and of the people who work there. My goal is to show how the institution's person-centered approach to transcultural psychiatry, its clinical organization, and its practices are deeply intertwined with its historical foundations and the personalities of the people who work there. In particular, I address ambiguities around the institution's positioning as both a voluntary association with strong moral mandates (Association Françoise et Eugène Minkowski) and a public health structure (Centre Minkowska). I argue that it operates as a production site of the state and is constrained by both its mission and its budget.

HISTORY OF CENTRE MINKOWSKA

Although refugees poured into France following World War II, few institutional centers were equipped with services to address their psychological distress. One that did was the Tiomkine Clinic, founded during World War II in the ninth arrondissement of Paris, where psychiatrist Eugène Minkowski offered consultations.

Eugène Minkowski and his wife, psychiatrist Françoise Minkowska, are not considered well-known historical figures, although they gained prominence within French psychiatry and psychopathology. Both studied and worked in Zurich with Eugen Bleuler, the first clinician to identify the concept of schizophrenia. In their early careers, Eugène and Françoise contributed to our understanding of that disorder before moving to Paris at the beginning of World War I, after Eugène signed up to become a doctor in the French army.

Between the world wars, Minkowski was involved in an international charity for poor Jewish children called *Union Oeuvre de Secours aux Enfants*. When France was divided during World War II, he committed to the resistance in the northern zone, including by setting up a clandestine network to place children in non-Jewish families. In the wake of World War II, Eugène and his family were arrested in their home, but with help from powerful friends, they avoided deportation. After this, Eugène launched a mental health consultation service, offering patients a form of care that acknowledged their particular life histories and provided services in their native languages. At the time, most of his patients were refugees from Eastern Europe.

When more refugees arrived from Central Europe, Eugène asked another psychiatrist, Dr. Joseph Fursay-Fusswerck, and a psychologist, Mrs. Kahn Dreyfus, to join him. In 1952, their clinic became funded by the SSAE (Service social d'aide aux émigrants). From the beginning, in order to facilitate refugees' access to the clinic and the effectiveness of clinical encounters, their consultations were open to adults and children and were offered in German, Russian, and Polish. Instead of using translators, patients were referred to psychiatrists of the same geographic and linguistic origin. In 1950, the Tiomkine Clinic created two additional consultation departments, one for Portuguese workers and the other for Hungarian refugees.

With continued immigration, the members of Minkowski's clinic decided a service welcoming all non-French-speaking patients should be created. Since the SSAE lacked the funds to support such an endeavor, Minkowski created the Association of Friends of Françoise Minkowska in 1962 so that funds could be raised to guarantee the center's pursuit of clinical activities and to purchase a larger building on the same street. An agreement was later signed with the Seine Mental Hygiene Services, which would fund the clinic thereafter. At Eugène Minkowski's request, the clinic was dedicated to his wife, who had passed away in 1950, and was named Centre Minkowska. In 1972, Eugène Minkowski died. The status of the association was modified in 1975 and renamed Association Françoise et Eugène Minkowski.

As immigration flows to France diversified, so did the center's clinical activity, which became organized around geographic and linguistic departments. Offices were spread over three different floors of the new building: the ground floor housed the North Africa and Asia departments, the first floor included administrative services, and the second floor was dedicated to the remaining department, which addressed the needs of migrants from Turkey, sub-Saharan Africa (referred to as *Afrique noire*), Portuguese-speaking countries, Spanish-speaking countries, and Central Europe. From Centre Minkowska's foundation, the clinical expertise of its staff focused not on culture per se but on life experiences, such as exile and related traumas, and their approach to mental illness was based on a universalistic model of mental health rather than a culturalist one. In fact, Eugène Minkowski and Swiss psychiatrist Ludwig Binswanger were the first to develop a phenomenological approach to psychiatry focused on the person's lived experience rather than searching for symptoms of mental distress. In that perspective, Minkowski strongly supported an anthropological approach to psychiatry and psychology. Influenced by the works of German philosopher Edmund Husserl and French philosopher Henri Bergson, Minkowski was convinced that "the mental syndrome is no longer for us a simple association of symptoms, but the expression of a profound and characteristic modification of the entire human personality" (quoted in Granger 1999, 107). Although Minkowski's approach to mental health was not called this at the time, he had already developed the global, person-centered approach that drives the center today.

In 1985, the center underwent a major status change and officially joined the public hospital system. For a while, this did not affect its clinical framework. As Marie Jo Bourdin—the current co-director of the center—told me, clinicians were

attached to their geocultural *équipes* (teams). During the 1980s, the right to cultural difference was legitimated through socialist president François Mitterand's
pro-immigrant discourse, which encouraged this type of organization. Although
the critique directed at Tobie Nathan's culturalist approach to mental health care
had negatively affected the center, its staff felt strongly attached to their humanist
roots and objectives—despite their geocultural clinical organization. They
expressed this directly through a letter sent to French newspaper *Le Monde* in 1996,
in response to an interview with Tobie Nathan in which he contended that his
consultation was the first of its kind to specifically cater to immigrants. The letter
from the Minkowska Centre corrected this error in the genealogy of specialized
mental health care, but it also refuted—in a quite satirical tone—Nathan's description of Centre Minkowska as a clinic that offered only a translated form of psychiatry: "According to him [Tobie Nathan], there are categories of patients for
whom *translated psychiatry* is useful: eastern Europeans, Russians, Polish, Italians
and Spaniards. And then, there are the others: for example, North Africans, who
are certainly a little more foreign than other foreigners. As for black Africans, let's
not even mention them. They must be a little more foreign than the foreigners
who are more foreign than other foreigners" (*Le Monde* 1996; my translation, ital-
ics in the original). The letter continues, identifying differences between
Nathan's and Centre Minkowska's clinical approaches:

> We learned that no patient is more foreign to us than another, and that is why we
> do not prevent any clinician from seeing the same patients we see. We do not pre-
> vent them from thinking about the Other [capitalization in original], nor to meet
> him, despite their cultural differences. Our main contribution is precisely to favor
> that encounter. We are not held up as experts simply on the basis that we speak
> the same language or that we are from the same culture. We are not even sure that
> one individual may ever be from the same culture as another, since as we leave our
> patient the freedom to translate—and this is how we construe the act of
> translation—his culture in his own, singular fashion, we realized that it was being
> progressively reinvented, and that he may need to distance [himself] from it, just
> as he may want to rely on it. We are not the ones who should assign him [our
> patient] to it [his culture] against his will, according to the representation we our-
> selves have of his culture. That is to say, we explicitly avoid the attitude adopted
> by Tobie Nathan, which consists in "testing a theory" on patients. (*Le Monde* 1996;
> my translation)

Despite this public position, Marie Jo recalled that the approach of some clinicians at the time was quite culturalist, and she often joked that you almost needed
a passport to cross clinical departments.

Over time, physical changes facilitated the center's transition to a new clinical
approach. In 1999, it moved to a new space in the seventeenth arrondissement of

Paris, where it is still located. While the geocultural organization of the clinic persisted, the office space was much smaller, and the physical divisions that existed in the ninth arrondissement location disappeared. At that point, the center's general director, Christophe Paris; the assistant director, Marie-Jo Bourdin; and the head of the medical committee, Dr. Rachid Bennegadi, began to collaborate on a plan to revamp the center's approach. Their objectives were to move beyond the lens of culture as the only approach to therapy with migrants and to rethink the center's past practice of systematically matching patients and clinicians. In this context, Dr. Bennegadi suggested clinical medical anthropology as a productive framework within therapy settings (Rostirolla and Wadoux 2017).

Clinical medical anthropology is not a therapeutic approach like psychoanalysis, cognitive behavioral therapy, or gestalt therapy, but it offers a broad framework that structures health-care delivery, within which any therapeutic approach could be applied. Dr. Bennegadi also meant to use it as a way to actively consider the role of cultural representations—as expressed by patients and clinicians—in mental health disorders. Within a clinical medical anthropology framework, the objective is to lead clinicians to think systemically about both health-care settings and interactions. To do so, Dr. Bennegadi and his colleagues borrowed conceptually from the clinical model that anthropologists Arthur Kleinman, Leon Eisenberg, and Byron Good (1978) developed to identify the confrontation of multiple explanatory models within clinical settings. Explanatory models refer to different understandings of a sickness episode and its relevant treatment by those engaged in the clinical process (the patient, the patient's family, a physician, a healer, and so on). The clinical model prioritizes identifying different social representations of illness, disease, and sickness that affect the provision of health care. By doing so, clinicians can better recognize that illness and care are embedded in social worlds, that their own clinical categories are cultural constructions, and that the clinician-patient interaction and the disease/illness experience are shaped by social determinants that must be considered when delivering care (Kleinman 1980).

By adopting a clinical medical anthropology (AMC) framework, the center's directors intended to avoid using any kind of narrow, culture-based framework for mental health care and to underscore the relevance of cultural aspects "as one element of care, not as the main analytical grid" (Bennegadi 1996, 445). While the center's directors do not expect clinicians to master anthropological theory, they hope that they will become more reflexive about common explanatory models—particularly biomedical classifications—that may overlook cultural aspects of their own and patients' representations of illness. The clinical medical anthropology framework also encourages general practitioners and clinicians—regardless of their theoretical orientation (psychoanalysis, psychotherapy)—to focus on providing the most appropriate diagnosis or referral. In this way, the new approach at the center is less about clinicians being from the same origin as the patient and more about "the issue of the universality of psychopathology" (Bennegadi 1996, 445). To put it simply, depression can be diagnosed across cultures, but its expression will vary from one culture to another, following local norms and representations. As a result, any clinician trained in the AMC approach can work with a patient from any cultural origin as long as she or he is able to practice the gymnastics of starting from the particular expression of distress to find the universal psychopathological root. Finally, the AMC framework "respects the French public health system's philosophy of health care access as a common/universal right (*droit commun*)" (Bennegadi 1996, 445), which the center's directors consider a core value of the institution. While other frameworks may respect this notion, clinical medical anthropology was specifically founded on that value. Despite the directors' articulation of this new model, the challenge for the center rests with health professionals' willingness to broaden their theoretical framework, "not through a magical process, but through professional training" (Bennegadi 1996, 445).

Institutionalizing AMC

The opportunity for this kind of framework transition manifested during the accreditation process set by the Health Authority Administration (HAS, Haute autorité de santé) in 1999. The process, inspired by American and Canadian models of health-care management (HAS 2017), focused on patient therapeutic itineraries and encouraged health institutions' responsibility in health provision. The HAS objectives were threefold: to provide management methods and tools that ensure quality and security in health care, to respond to users' transparency requirements, and to promote health-care reporting and regulation by ensuring health-care quality (HAS 2017). The first line of accreditation included promoting HAS's objectives and familiarizing institutions with the measures they should take to improve quality of care. During the second version of the certification, launched in 2005, institutions were evaluated, with the aim of identifying and evaluating "best practices" in relation to the institution's missions, health field, and targeted populations, thus "reinforcing the medicalization of this process" (HAS 2017). With the help of HAS experts, each institution was to develop its own indicators, which would serve as the basis for their accreditation examination. From my fieldwork experience within other French health settings, such as hospitals, I can attest that this accreditation process requires a tremendous amount of work and energy and is a source of great tension for months prior to the experts' examination.

For Centre Minkowska, the accreditation process began in 2005 and would not be completed until 2007. In order to implement their new AMC framework while also obtaining HAS accreditation, Centre Minkowska staff had to transform the way they organized their consultations. Whereas patients were dispatched to therapists according to their spoken language and culture of origin in the center's original model, administrative secretaries were no longer allowed to elicit such information or use it as a basis for therapy referral; consequently, the section on dividing consultations into geographic zones was removed from the center's patient information form. Although language has remained a criterion for determining therapist designation, it is no longer necessarily based on a patient's first language but may be based on a language the patient and therapist have in common (e.g., English). Clinicians are now trained to work with interpreters, which makes internal referrals considerably more flexible and less stigmatizing. Over the past decade, Centre Minkowska has moved toward an approach that is more person-centered, transcultural, and based on the clinical medical anthropology framework. With the accreditation process obtained in 2007, the AMC framework was recognized by HAS as a "best practice," which legitimated it both within the public health field and at Centre Minkowska. A few years later, the framework lost its social relevance within HAS, and "cultural competence" progressively replaced "clinical medical anthropology" when speaking of best mental health care practice.

Changing Organizational Practices, Closing the Travel Agency

For many years, the center's patient files were all on paper, with a sheet collecting sociodemographic information, such as the patient's living situation (with parents, with a partner, at a shelter, alone, with children), any legal protection or supervision (legal surveillance, hospital supervision, tutor supervision), forms of social assistance (disability, unemployment, social security stipends), place of external referral if applicable, school status, and professional status. Initially, this sheet had a space to indicate the patient's geographic area of origin within seven major categories: Africa/Indian Ocean/Caribbean, Spain and Spanish-speaking countries, Portugal and Portuguese-speaking countries, Central and Eastern Europe, Turkey, Asia, and North Africa. Secretaries then had the option of assigning patients to a therapist who specialized in a particular geographic area. Files were organized accordingly into geolinguistic *armoires* (filing cabinets), casting patients into categories that related cultural belonging to very broad linguistic regions.

This model of organizing the clinic became increasingly problematic as center staff made efforts to dissociate from the bad press around Nathan's culture-specific model of mental health care. While it was socially acceptable at the time for mental health provision to continue labeling itself as culturally competent and to address the needs of migrant populations in the name of health-care access for all, it was no longer acceptable for clinics to refer to specific ethnic groups or to formally triage patients according to their place of origin. While that form of organization held sway during Minkowska's early years, the center's mission and structural organization began to change: the visible needed to be made invisible.

Central to this process of change was the reorganization of how the center collected information about patients, organized its filing system, and assigned patients to therapists. As a result of the accreditation process in the mid-2000s, such changes were made—among them the removal of the geographic area indicator on the patient information form. When I arrived at Centre Minkowska for my dissertation fieldwork in 2007, it was precisely the moment when this major transition was taking place. The institutional-level changes triggered much resistance among staff members. I remember a conversation I had with Marie-Jo at that time, which perfectly illustrates that resistance to change. That day, she talked to me about one of her greatest burdens, which was to manage the "old" secretarial team, referring to three secretaries, two of whom had been working at the center for over twenty years. The descriptor was used not only to reference the secretaries' lengthy service at Minkowska but also to indirectly emphasize that the organization, institutional standing, and clinical framework of the center had shifted significantly during those past two decades. Accordingly, the center had gone through several changes, of which the most significant were its filing and referral practices. Conflicts at the center among the staff often related to internal resistance or lack of adaptation to such changes. As we carried on our conversation, Marie-Jo suddenly interrupted her sentence, paying attention to the voice of one of the "old-team" secretaries answering a phone call in the office next door. I started listening as well, trying to understand what had suddenly caught Marie-Jo's attention. The secretary, Andrée, was questioning her phone interlocutor: "Camara . . . Camara . . . is that Soninke? Where is the patient from? [Pause] And what language does he speak? [Pause] I'm going to try to see if I have any available appointment with Dr. S. then." Andrée had spent her entire career as a medical secretary at Minkowska. Close to retirement, she did not look favorably on the organizational changes that the certification process entailed.

Following Andrée's phone response, Marie-Jo rolled her eyes and said, "See what I have to deal with, every day? Imagine if the public health evaluation team heard that one day! This could cost us our public health accreditation! I keep telling them not to do this anymore, openly asking details about patient's ethnic background over the phone. This is not how we do things anymore! I'm telling you, I can't wait until they all retire and I no longer have to deal with this!"

Marie-Jo then explained how she, Christophe Paris, and Dr. Bennegadi painstakingly prepared the staff for the 2006 audits, which included having the secretaries practice how to answer the phone. They could no longer just triage patients by asking questions about their ethnic group or their place of origin, and there was no obligation to refer a patient to Dr. Sarr—one of the two clinicians of sub-Saharan African origin working at the center—simply because the patient was of African origin. Marie-Jo insisted that the center no longer wanted to be perceived that way: "Really, their only potential concern should be about patients' spoken language. It's hard for the secretaries to understand, though, and honestly, they just don't put much effort into it. They're close to retiring, and they won't change their ways." She told me how she kept explaining to the secretaries the AMC framework, the importance of finding a middle ground between culture as all-encompassing in health-care delivery, which ultimately leads to patients' stigmatization, and culture-blind care, which leads to ethnocentrism. Marie-Jo's comments made it clear that even a seemingly minor policy change in managing patients' files created compliance difficulties for some staff members, which led to tensions between them and others, who found the same changes more important and easier to manage.

The changes to which Marie-Jo referred were logical within the center's AMC framework and within the French public health system's shift to provide health-care access for everyone, regardless of national origin or legal status. As Marie-Jo likes to put it each time she narrates the history of the center to visitors or guests: "We closed the travel agency"! In the center's everyday practice, though, some secretaries continued to dispatch patients to therapists based on their culture of origin or spoken languages. This disparity between institutional discourse on organizing principles and everyday clinical practice unsurprisingly triggered internal misunderstandings and conflict, especially among older staff members, who negotiated the institutional changes less easily. Shortly after Marie-Jo complained about the "old" team's behavior, I started research into patients' files, housed in the secretaries' office, and spoke about the same issue with Andrée.

I began, "So, I just learned about the auditing process for the accreditation and about the small changes that came along with that in the referring system. . . . That must have been stressful for you all."

In low tones, which I suspected she used to avoid being overheard by senior staff, Andrée replied, "This is just ridiculous. Marie-Jo keeps being on our case about not asking details on the patients' origins over the phone, but how else would we go about and organize referrals here? I've served as a secretary for Dr. Sarr and Mr. Kouassi for years now." She pointed to the clinicians' respective appointment books, piled on her desk, and continued: "It has always made sense so far that we refer patients of African origin to them. After all, they do understand the culture and they do speak the same language as the patient's sometimes. That's what people presumably call us for. To find someone to talk to who will understand."

I nodded at Andrée's comments, reminded about what happened after I was given research permission to go through patients' files: the senior staff sent me to Andrée as the secretary "in charge of African patients." She had directed me to the filing cabinet behind her, where she noted that the files on African patients were grouped. When I began my doctoral research, each filing cabinet was organized according to patients' geographic area of origin. During research, though, I witnessed the center's transition from using geocultural *armoires* to a unified, numerical filing system. This symbolic first step toward a new approach was followed by another in the summer of 2009: during significant renovation work, the divisions that separated secretaries' offices—a remnant of past institutional organization around geocultural lines—were removed. Amid the reorganization of office space, a single open space was designated for all secretaries as the welcome area. The room next to it housed all patient files, now organized in alphabetical order. In 2017, this organizational system was integrated even further when the center switched to a computerized patient file program.

TRANSCULTURAL PRACTICE AND PRACTITIONERS

Today, Centre Minkowska is identified by the public health system as both a *centre médico-psychologique* (mental health center) and an *établissement privé d'intérêt collectif* (private institution of collective interest). In the public health system, it is affiliated with the Fédération des établissements hospitaliers et d'assistance privés à but non lucratif (federation of nonprofit private hospital and assistance institutions). Unlike other mainstream CMPs, the center does not serve a limited geographical sector. Because it was founded as an association promoting the mental health of migrants and not directly as a public institution linked to a district hospital, it may receive patients from across the greater Paris region (Ile-de-France).[2] Consultations are free, which eases the financial burden of health-care access. Minkowska's 2016 activity report highlights that "consultations offered to immigrants and refugees are the same as for any other person in France, regardless of origin" (Association Françoise et Eugène Minkowski 2017, 11). This policy remains faithful to the original vision of the clinic's founders though having been adapted to fit the organization of public health care in contemporary France.

In 2016, Centre Minkowska treated 1,618 patients. Among these, 731 were new patients. That number has steadily increased, and almost half reside in Paris. These patients are referred by various agencies, including—in order of importance by number of referrals—social services, public health institutions, general practitioners, other associations, schools, and justice institutions. As I will show, motives for referrals are highly variable and not always clearly articulated. The center's logic for mental health-care delivery and the contours of its clinical expertise are defined in its 2016 activity report in relation to three common scenarios:

1. The referred person does not share the same language as the therapist. When there is no language in common between the two, then linguistic and cultural interpreting is used. This allows the consultation to take place, the potential disorder to be identified, and, if necessary, a diagnosis to be made, along with a therapeutic proposition.
2. The referred person and the therapist have a language in common, in which case there is no need for an interpreter, but communication may still be challenging when the person expresses suffering by relying on his or her own cultural representations and social references for mental disorder. In this specific situation, all therapists in the institutions are trained to take into consideration

cultural representations and social references (which constitute an explanatory model). They may thus acknowledge their own representations of mental disorders, identify psychiatric or psychological categories of distress, and better understand what the person expresses (illness).

3. When the referral is for a couple or a family who does not speak the same language as the therapist's, then it is preferable to rely on cultural mediation. The difference between an interpreter and a cultural mediator lies in the fact that a mediator not only has interpreting skills but also masters the clinical medical anthropology approach. (Association Françoise et Eugène Minkowski 2017, 13; my translation)

In later text, the activity report notes, "These three situations prove that the therapeutic framework is perfectly compatible with public healthcare, by not culturally assigning nor stigmatizing the person. In other words, in the context of best practice, it is not necessary to ethnicize the therapeutic framework in order to provide care to someone." Progressively, Centre Minkowska has opted for a cultural competence approach, which is defined on its website as the integration of three dimensions within clinical practice: the cultural, which highlights the importance of attention to patients' cultural representations of suffering; the linguistic, which includes working with professional interpreters when there is no language in common between the therapist and the patient; and the social, which takes into account social determinants directly affecting individuals' mental health, such as lack of housing, unemployment, or irregular administrative status. Overall, the center's clinical activity has increased, but its logistical and financial means have remained the same. I describe the tensions that result from this scenario in later chapters in this book.

The Team

The current professional team at Minkowska is relatively small. A sense of familiarity exists between colleagues, which influences professional relationships. The direction committee consists of Christophe Paris, the director general; Marie-Jo Bourdin, the assistant director; and Dr. Rachid Bennegadi, the head of the medical committee. These three have worked together for over two decades. Marie-Jo was the first of the three to be hired at the center, and she has witnessed its many changes over time. She arrived in 1982 and was employed as the social worker for two departments: Portugal and Portuguese-speaking people and Africa/Indian Ocean/Caribbean. For Marie-Jo, working at Minkowska was an opportunity to integrate two professional interests: community psychiatry and her desire to work for the French branch of the SSAE: "When I arrived at Minkowska, I was one of the rare French persons 'of origin' [i.e., white French background] to work there, which raised suspicion and sometimes made my work difficult."

Dr. Rachid Bennegadi arrived at the center in 1985. He had migrated from Algeria after independence to complete his residency in cardiology in Paris. Because of degree disparities between Algeria and France, which negated some of the credentials of his prior training, he switched to psychiatry. While completing his residency in that field, he obtained a graduate degree in anthropology. Dr. Bennegadi practiced psychiatry in various hospital settings in Paris, including Hôpital Necker, where he met French psychiatrist Yves Pelicier, with whom he was able to share his frustrations about being identified as "the Arab doctor." For example, after a few months working at Necker, Dr. Bennegadi realized that he was only being referred patients from North Africa. He told me that when he had asked the medical secretaries why this was the case, they had said that "it made sense" and that it was "easier" that way. Dr. Bennegadi argued that while they may have been right for language purposes, he also wanted to see "other" patients. This would be the beginning of a career-long struggle for Dr. Bennegadi. When he arrived at Minkowska, he quickly upset his colleagues. Marie-Jo told me how even she felt annoyed at how readily he wanted to revoke the geocultural basis of consultations. For a long time, Dr. Bennegadi worked in relative isolation.

Christophe Paris arrived at Centre Minkowska in 1997. Not yet thirty, he was just beginning his professional career as a public health administrator, having attended a school of management for health and social institutions. Given that he was considerably younger (by two decades) and less professionally experienced than Marie-Jo or Dr. Bennegadi, it must not have always been easy for him to assert his authority. However, he managed to build a very collegial relationship with them, and when I met the three in 2007, I was struck by their warm collaboration. They would often stay late to debrief and work together on media training tools for the AMC approach. Although Christophe does not appear much as a protagonist in this ethnography, he was pivotal—along with Marie-Jo and Dr. Bennegadi—in helping transform the identity of Centre Minkowska and its organization.

The other colleagues I will introduce in this book are central actors in the organization of MEDIACOR meetings. Like me, they were hired more recently. Among them we will meet two psychiatrists, Dr. Smaïl Cheref—introduced earlier in the book, and Dr. Maria Vittoria Carlin. Dr. Cheref met Marie-Jo and Dr. Bennegadi when the two co-organized a workshop, called Shared Perspectives, at Hôpital Sainte-Anne. Smaïl Cheref worked in a general psychiatry unit, and he was interested in Centre Minkowska's AMC approach, likely finding that discussions of cultural difference echoed his own trajectory and experience as a migrant from Algeria. He regularly attended the workshop and served as a discussant on several occasions. The center was looking for a part-time psychiatrist at the time, and Dr. Cheref was interested in the position; he joined the team in 2011. Dr. Carlin arrived a few years later, in 2015, although she worked at the center as a trainee before being hired as a psychiatrist. She is a tall woman, with short chestnut-colored hair. She is very dynamic and often speaks with a smile on her face. She was born and raised in Italy but left after her residency to work abroad on humanitarian interventions in Palestine and Morocco, after which she spent a few years in Spain volunteering for Médecins du monde in order to attend to the mental health of undocumented migrants. In those humanitarian work contexts, she claims to have found a vocation. She was told of Centre Minkowska's work by a partner institution in Barcelona, the SAPPIR center.

Verthançia, a social worker, and Audrey, a nurse, are among the youngest on the team. Verthançia, hired in 2013, was born in the Democratic Republic of Congo, and her family migrated to France when she was two years old. Now, in her early thirties, Verthançia is petite in size but assertive in character. I often joke with her that she is the most fashionable person I know, as she always sports the latest clothing styles and is not afraid of bold colors. Because of her background, she says she has always been interested in working in a transcultural context. She knew of Centre Minkowska by reputation. One of her close friends had been the center's previous social worker, and when she left the center, she recommended Verthançia to Marie-Jo. Audrey, on the other hand, had not heard of Centre Minkowska, and she had just completed her nursing degree when she saw a job posting for a medical secretary at the center. It was close to the summer season and she figured that she could take a temporary job at the center while waiting for a nursing position to open up at a nearby hospital or clinic. She was formally hired as a nurse a few months later and charged with managing the medical secretaries and triaging incoming referrals. Audrey—a slender, short-haired blonde in her mid-twenties—is a very private person. She regularly works in tandem with Verthançia.

Minkowska's Staff and Time Commitments

Within the center, there are three different but overlapping fields of activity: the clinic and the teaching and research department, both directed by Dr. Bennegadi, and the professional training department, directed by Marie-Jo. Few clinicians work in the clinic full time. Dr. Bennegadi is present most often, working at the center in the afternoons from Monday through Thursday, and all day on Friday. Dr. Carlin, who speaks Italian, Spanish, and English, works at the clinic two days a week, and Dr. Cheref, who speaks Arabic and Kabyle (spoken in Algeria), works at Minkowska two and a half days a week. In 2017, Dr. Cheref was appointed head of the medical commission known as CME (Commission médicale d'Etablissement).[3] The center has three other psychiatrists, but they are less involved: Dr. Sarr, who speaks Wolof (spoken in Senegal), works one day a week; Dr. Hodza, who speaks Serbian, works one day a week; and Dr. Luong, who speaks Vietnamese and English, works one and a half days a week.

The nine psychologists who work at Centre Minkowska also distribute their time unequally: Ms. Vasquez, who speaks Portuguese, and Ms. Rostirolla, who speaks Italian, both work two days a week. Mr. Kouassi, who speaks Baoulé, and Ms. Ayouch, who speaks Arabic, both work one day a week. The remaining five psychologists each work half a day per week: Ms. Penpe, who speaks Turkish; Ms. Mendieta, who speaks Spanish; Mr. Guberina, who speaks Serbian and English; Mr. Barzin, who speaks Farsi and Dari; and Mr. Meliz, who speaks Russian and Georgian.

The full-time staff is composed of two medical secretaries in charge of welcoming patients. Audrey, the nurse, sees patients on their first appointment and is in charge of screening referrals in preparation for staff meetings (MEDIACOR); Verthançia, the social worker, assists patients with issues ranging from medical coverage to housing issues and legal paperwork, attends patient evaluations, and participates in joint-therapy sessions between social workers and clinicians. There is also an accountant; a marketing manager in charge of training programs; and me, a medical anthropologist and psychotherapist who coordinates teaching and research activities and receives patients under the supervision of Dr. Bennegadi. Most of us who work at Centre Minkowska do so out of professional interest, a sense of social justice, and personal engagement with issues around immigration. Although it is well known among those working within the Parisian public health system, it is a small clinic and salaries are low; in other words, this is not a place people seek out for career advancement. In that respect, Centre Minkowska, to use Paul Brodwin's (2013) characterization of community psychiatry in the United States, is a moralized workplace.

Transcultural Clinicians: Migration, Reflexivity, and the Professional Project

Throughout this ethnography, as I have already done with Marie-Jo, I provide portraits of professional actors at Centre Minkowska. I do so in order to delve into colleagues' personal ethos and assess how this ethos intersects with their professional goals, ultimately to trace the moral processes at work in the activities of the clinic.

Within transcultural psychiatry, the ability of clinicians to empathize with their patients has been linked to ideas about their expertise. In France, the people who lead institutional practice on specialized mental health care for migrants tend to have a personal history with immigration, and many are migrants themselves (Larchanché 2010; Moro et al. 2004). Because of this, these leaders often have strong personal convictions that influence their professional endeavors. Beyond expertise in languages other than French, their authority is buttressed by their life trajectories; they are familiar with the hardships that migrants endure. This may sound like a relativist assertion, but in the case of transcultural practice, an expert who is also a migrant wields powerful credentials in terms of symbolic representation within institutions.

Dr. Bennegadi's childhood experience in colonized Algeria instilled in him an identity dilemma: he perceived himself as both Arab Algerian and French. In the life history he wrote for me, he recalled:

> It was not clear to me, especially as a child, that I had to absorb at a young age the paradox of being a French citizen, as explained by my French teachers, and simultaneously understand the terrible repression against people of my Arab ethnic group who were fighting against French colonialism in Algeria, Morocco, and Tunisia during my youth. . . . My father would try to help my siblings and me comprehend this apparent paradox of allegiances by explaining that we Algerians had nothing against French civilization, but we would never accept it under pressure and intimidation. It took me years of both humiliation and gratification to resolve this identity dilemma. Eventually, I was able to defend both the poetry of Victor Hugo and the extraordinary stories of the golden age of Islam. Both were transmitted by my father, who I came to realize had decided to leave to me and my siblings the opportunity to evolve our own self-image as both Arab Algerians and French.
>
> My first real cultural shock was when I discovered in 1962, when Algeria gained independence from France, that all my college friends were gone; they'd felt forced, by the intense turmoil of the years leading to independence, to identify themselves definitively as French citizens and return to mainland France, "the metropole," despite their families having lived for several generations as French Algerians. That is when I suddenly realized that I too would one day have to make a similar choice between identifying myself as either Algerian or French and could no longer be viewed by others, or view myself, as what would now be called a "bi-cultural" person.

Dr. Bennegadi's case is particularly fascinating because it portrays the intricacy of the issue of cultural allegiance under colonialism. The sense of dual cultural belonging, easily negotiated by Dr. Bennegadi as a child, was lost when he came to France, where he felt that he was always being regarded as an Arab.

Dr. Bennegadi's decision to introduce clinical medical anthropology to Centre Minkowska, a model that necessitates seeing beyond personal cultural identification within professional endeavors, thus resulted from his own existential struggles around identity. Even before immigrating to France, though, he experienced confrontations between multiple worldviews. After completing his medical degree in Oran, he was drafted into military service in the Algerian Sahara and worked with the Bedouin population of that region. For two years he ran a local hospital, operating it in the difficult sociopolitical climate of postwar Algeria and navigating cultural difference. In his life history, he writes:

> I soon discovered that I had to take on responsibilities and make decisions I was not prepared for, and I also had to cope with different conceptions of health and

illness among people in the same country I grew up in, who I presumed shared the same cultural background and values as I did. But I realized every day how large the conceptual gap between me and my Bedouin patients was: I had to explain to them the causes of infectious diseases, as well as psychiatric problems. In order to convince them to accept modern medicine's treatment methods, I had to learn how to negotiate an acceptable treatment plan, integrating my scientific knowledge and skills with traditional beliefs in illness causation and treatment regimens. I learned how to integrate the biomedical value system I learned in medical school with traditional Bedouin magical beliefs without losing my mind, or my status as a doctor trying to do my best for the sake of my patients' well-being.

This experience is what led Dr. Bennegadi to pursue a dual degree in anthropology and psychiatry, under the supervision of François Raveau at EHESS in Paris, Georges Devos at UC Berkeley, and Yves Pélicier at Hôpital Necker in Paris. In 1983, he received a Fulbright grant to study "culture and personality" at the Institute of Personality Assessment and Research at the University of California, Berkeley. During his stay in California, he participated in systemic therapy meetings at the Palo Alto school with Paul Watzlawick, and became familiar with the clinical medical anthropology framework that later influenced his approach at Minkowska:

> That was a major learning and growth experience for me. Once again, I had to cope with a very different educational system and different values than that in which I had grown up in French Algeria and in France. That experience, and my need to cope with the conceptual changes inherent in adapting to living and studying in California, changed my way of thinking, just as anthropology had opened my mind and my sphere of interest to ethics, philosophy and cybernetics. Back in France after four months in California, I took an active part in introducing clinical medical anthropology in French cultural studies, which seemed to me at that time to be very ethnocentrically biased. I don't know just which aspects of my life experience up to that time gave me this feeling, but I did understand that changing culturally engendered thought patterns would require a sustained effort over many years, and I decided to commit myself to that endeavor.

Again, this reflexive narrative illustrates a direct correlation between this clinician's life trajectory and his understanding of the relevance of both the universal and the particular in the therapeutic context—and beyond. This is key to understanding clinical medical anthropology as it developed at Minkowska and its related cultural competence approach: although individuals express psychological distress or psychiatric disorders in unique ways—based on their individual life history, personality type, context, and cultural representations—psychopathology is universal. Rachid Bennegadi developed a more clearly universalistic clinical framework because his personal and academic experiences directly placed the universal and the particular in tension, resulting in his emphasis on the universal imperative in cultural competence. As he often says, "The disorder is universal, only its clothing is cultural (*l'habillage est culturel*)." In line with Eugène Minkowski, Dr. Bennegadi often calls on a phenomenological approach to the clinical encounter and to the illness experience. As I show later, he regularly invites students, through self-reflexive practice, to develop this approach in their evaluation of patient referrals. He is a firm believer that the future of transcultural psychiatry lies in the development of social psychiatry as a discipline that focuses on stigma and the complex dynamics of belonging in a global context, rather than on cultural identity per se.

MEDIACOR AND PERFORMING AMC

Another major transition in the life of the institution occurred with the creation of a work unit called *Dispositif de Médiation, Accueil, et Orientation* (MEDIACOR) in January 2009. This interdisciplinary work group was founded in response to the center's increasing number of patient referrals—many seemingly unjustified or misdirected—and being unable to meet the demand. The goal of MEDIACOR is to analyze incoming referrals in ways that secretaries, who usually make the appointments, do not have the time or the qualifications to do. Its task is to contact referring institutions when their referrals are deemed problematic—that is, when it is unclear what role Minkowska as a specialized mental health center should play in accommodating the referred individual. Before Audrey arrived and was placed in charge of welcoming patients, Marie-Jo and Dr. Cheref would evaluate referrals twice a week and contact referring institutions themselves. As I illustrate, when referrals are clearly misdirected, the group's task is to find an alternative, more appropriate structure to assume responsibility for the individual. The group's goal is to compile and analyze data on both problematic and successful referrals, so guidelines and new policies may be implemented as a way for the center to improve the referral process and ultimately improve patient care. This is where my work as a practicing anthropologist is most productive. I like to think the conversations I had with the center's professionals during my doctoral research indirectly inspired the creation of such a unit.

Another factor that certainly influenced the creation of MEDIACOR was the HAS certification process, which started in 2005. MEDIACOR acts in part as a tool for the evaluation of professional practices (EPP) by analyzing the relevance of referrals. The analysis that started at that time has shown that response delays exceeded three months, which often caused patients to cancel appointments or simply not show up. It also documented secretarial work overload caused by the ambiguity of referrals, therapists being overbooked, and long appointment delays. In reaction to the team's analysis of the center's intake processes, the MEDIACOR unit was created. Its objectives were to devise responses that are fluid and adapted to so-called complex or time-consuming referrals, create a shared appointment calendar for all therapists, formalize an intake document to help secretaries' decision making, formalize intake forms for MEDIACOR professionals, and reorganize secretarial work. The unit also participated in another EPP, this one an evaluation of the main types of health pathologies and problems the center addresses. It was initiated after Dr. Bennegadi, Marie-Jo, and Christophe pointed out that the procedures used for follow-up of migrant patients, organized on the basis of a therapists' linguistic or cultural skills alone, no longer fit with the AMC approach. This time, Centre Minkowska engaged in the EPP process to improve health-care provision to migrant populations within a framework based on clinical medical anthropology. The institution compared its care provision methods to other European and international clinical approaches. This analysis was carried out by the same team in conjunction with the transcultural psychiatry department at McGill University in Montreal, Canada, which was led by Laurence Kirmayer and inspired by the work of the Cultural Consultation Services at the Jewish Hospital in Montreal, directed by Dr. Eric Jarvis. Suggestions for improvement from this second EPP included reorganizing health-care delivery around the concept of cultural competence, which would be interfaced by MEDIACOR; creating multimedia tools to allow for the transfer of skills in the field of clinical medical anthropology; and initiating or pursuing research collaboration with universities in Europe and abroad. These actions relied not only on clinical activities but on the formalization of professional training, research, and teaching.

PROMOTING "CULTURAL COMPETENCE": TEACHING AND TRAINING AT CENTRE MINKOWSKA

In the chapter, I have described the relevance of AMC and the cultural competence approach in the activities at Minkowska, but this discussion would not be complete without detailing Minkowska's teaching and professional training activities. In addition to working in MEDIACOR, my work as an applied medical anthropologist is most salient in teaching and training. When I joined Centre Minkowska as a professional, I felt some uneasiness when the directors assigned me the task of teaching cultural competence skills to social and health professionals in the continuing education program and in professional training sessions. At the time, Centre Minkowska's directors did not readily adhere to the concept. Because they had devoted so much time and energy to developing the AMC model as a way to distance the center from earlier culturalist approaches to mental health care, they initially understood cultural competence as another essentializing approach to cultural difference in the clinic. After many years of training and working with mental health professionals, I have realized that as social scientists, we sometimes overlook the needs and thought processes of these professionals in deference to those of their patients. The perspectives of many professionals with whom I work are initially narrow; I have heard countless totalizing questions, such as, "How do we deal with Africans?" During our training sessions, however, their perspectives expand and their uneasiness responding to difference comes to the fore. This provides an opportunity for such feelings to be explored through discussions around cultural competence.

Sarah Willen and Elizabeth Carpenter-Song (2013) have published a volume that responds to the almost unanimous critique of cultural competence within anthropology: that it relies on essentializing notions of "culture" and that its training framework ignores broader socioeconomic conditions that influence health (Castañeda 2010). However, I would argue that this is a narrow understanding of the framework: it is characterized simply as an exercise in reflecting on the relevance of culture for patients and clinicians. In contrast, the framework deployed at Centre Minkowska—through the pedagogical work of MEDIACOR, professional training sessions, and the university continuing education program—is a systemic approach to health care that takes into account patients' and clients' cultural representations as only one aspect among many that influence health provision (e.g., social determinants of health). The center's objective is not to train "cultural experts" but to train professionals to think systemically and identify structural vulnerabilities that affect patients (Quesada, Hart, and Bourgois 2011). The way the model is used at Minkowska addresses reducing inequalities in general, without implying that inequalities are experienced only by migrant populations. In this respect, our program addresses critiques of cultural competence in general (Metzl and Hansen 2014).

The program at Minkowska is first and foremost multidisciplinary. People who come to teach students are professors from medical specialties and the social sciences, health professionals across specialties and institution categories (hospitals, district-based clinics), professionals working at NGOs, and professionals from Centre Minkowska itself. The program was created in 1996 with Silla Consoli, a psychiatrist at Université Paris Descartes Medical School and head of the Liaison Psychiatry Service at Georges Pompidou European Hospital. The spectrum of themes tackled in the program is intentionally wide; the idea is to accommodate cross-institutional interests in cultural competence. Professionals who enroll in the program come from diverse backgrounds: some are students in anthropology and psychology; others are social workers, nurses, doctors, educators, and NGO leaders. Some instructors come from abroad. Courses take place approximately one day a month, and each day ends with the presentation of a clinical or social situation from the perspective of cultural competence or with the supervision of a students' thesis work.

The year starts with an introduction to cultural competence from a clinical medical anthropology perspective. Dr. Bennegadi and I teach these core classes, which shape and contextualize the rest of the year's activities. I give students a critical genealogy of the management of migrant populations in France and introduce them to the importance of paying attention to—and distancing themselves from—social representations. I also introduce medical anthropology from an evolutionary perspective, so students are better able to identify the epistemological obstacles anthropologists had to overcome to understand health as something that is socially produced (Baer, Singer, and Susser 1997; Kleinman, Das, and Lock 1997). I illustrate why health must be analyzed at the intersection of individual biography and social and physical-environmental contexts (Quesada, Hart, and Bourgois 2011). In another core class, I address acculturation processes, their impact on identity strategies, and their potentially related psychopathologies. I explain how terminology and the construction of social categories are critical for enabling professionals to reflect on how they relate to migrants (Castañeda 2010). Professor Laurence Kotobi, a medical anthropologist from Université Bordeaux 2, joins me in the course and addresses the construction of social categories, their logics, and their impact on differential medical access and treatment practices. She also highlights the gendered components of medical practices. Finally, the program addresses the importance of working with interpreters and of cultivating good communication in the provision of care.

An equally important skill covered in this cultural competence program is reflexivity and the capacity to decenter from one's professional training and personal convictions. To do this, I invite students to think critically about the term "expert" and what it conveys about certainty and definite knowledge, which are antithetical to cultural competence as we construe it. Guzder and Rousseau (2013) suggest that the notion of an expert supports the hegemony and standardization of medical and psychiatric knowledge. In contrast, our objective in the program follows transcultural psychiatrist Laurence Kirmayer's suggestion to "embrac[e] uncertainty as a path to competence" (2013, 365). In our model, we consider anxieties in the face of complexity, uncertainty, and difference to be both social and personal. We also consider challenges to the practice and acquisition of cultural competence in mental health care to be constrained by external and internal factors. External factors include France's unique ideological context and institutional environment, as I unveil in later chapters. They also include contemporary approaches to rationalizing and measuring expertise in health care—particularly those that lose sight of the human.

While these are important components of the program, not everyone who participates is open to engaging in decentering and reflexivity. Many have worked with migrants, worked abroad, or been exposed through reading or training or become otherwise familiar with sociological or anthropological perspectives on contemporary issues (Larchanché 2010). Often they leave the program with a more acute consciousness of the challenges lying before them, which can be a destabilizing experience. As one student told me at the end of the program, "I feel like I hit a reboot button. Cultural competence is about being de-programmed." This gaze-changing process affects professional and institutional practices: I have seen it increase professionals' critical-thinking skills and challenge the social categories through which these professionals view and understand their patients in general, not just migrants.

* * *

The institutional analysis of Centre Minkowska's evolution through successive paradigms of specialized mental health care highlights the challenges staff members face in maneuvering between humanist ethics of care, inherited from founding figure Eugène Minkowski, and two simultaneously constraining forces: the increasingly managerial logics of the health-care system, to which the center is subjected as a public health institution, and the larger societal dynamics that hinder health-care provision and social support to migrants in mainstream state institutions. Transcultural professionals at Minkowska are acutely aware of this ambiguity, as I have illustrated in relation to MEDIACOR. This very recognition allows them to critically reflect on clinical modalities in responding to potentially stigmatizing referrals, as I show in the following chapters.

PART II REFERRAL NARRATIVES AND ETHICAL DOUBLE BINDS

In the second part of this book, I explore how the need for a specialized form of mental health care for migrants has been discursively constructed in contemporary France through a range of stakeholders' motivations. In particular, I address obstacles invoked by state agents as motivations for their referrals to Centre Minkowska. During my fieldwork, I noticed their rationales tended to fall under two major categories: cultural or linguistic obstacles to care within mainstream institutions. At times, these obstacles were very real, but state agents also used these rationales as simple alibis to rid themselves of problematic situations. Sometimes referrals were motivated by structural obstacles related to a patient's precarious administrative status within government bureaucracy or to related constraints around institutional access and support. As I show in the following chapters, rationales around all obstacles tended to overlap—especially since structural obstacles are often attributed to cultural or linguistic difference.

In order to understand individual or institutional referrals and the moral subjectivities they express, I argue that referrals must be analyzed alongside broader moral economies that have influenced contemporary republican France. These include the state's anxious relationship to cultural difference, its history of hierarchizing populations during early industrial capitalism, colonization and the black slave trade (Mbembe 2016). In my analysis, I focus on representations of sub-Saharan migrants both because they have received particular attention recently from state institutions involved in the management of immigration and because they constitute a large proportion of the clientele presenting to specialized mental health centers. I show how nationwide political characterization of sub-Saharan migrants as culturally maladapted or socially deviant affects state agents' interpretation of their situations as pathological or requiring expert care. I pay particular attention to state agents' processes of differentiation based on locally intelligible linguistic practices, such as the use of code words that directly index cultural difference (e.g., the word *banlieue*, meaning "suburb," directly indexes a residential environment prone to social precarity and cultural diversity, a place where migrants are likely to live).

Through this analysis, I begin to identify the ethical double binds that are experienced by staff members at Centre Minkowska, and argue that such binds are related both to the center's ambiguous foundation as a public health institution and a voluntary association, and to the identification of its clinicians as cultural experts. I explore the ethical negotiations that derive from double-bind situations and how these influence mental health care experts' values, affects, judgments, and feelings.

3 · CULTURAL AND LINGUISTIC DIFFERENCE AS OBSTACLES TO CARE

Returning to Paris the summer of 2009, following my fieldwork, I was given the opportunity to attend an off-site consultation with Centre Minkowska. That day, we drove to a psychiatric hospital located in a southeastern suburb of Paris. I joined Marie-Jo and Salimata, a Wolof-Soninke-Bambara interpreter. We were to meet the patient, Mrs. Kouyate, and her husband—a middle-aged, first-generation migrant from Mali. Accompanied by a family elder, Mr. Kouyate had gone to Minkowska a few weeks earlier to discuss his wife with one of the center's psychiatrists.

Mrs. Kouyate had already been referred to Minkowska in 2006 by the staff of a maternity hospital in Paris. This had followed the home birth of her daughter, Sadio, during the thirty-fourth week of pregnancy. When the emergency services arrived on-site, Mrs. Kouyate was convinced that Sadio was dead. According to hospital professionals, Mrs. Kouyate had barely received any antenatal care. She was forty-one years old at the time, was not working, and had a temporary visa. It was her seventh pregnancy: two children had been born in Mali, two others had been born but died within forty-eight hours, and two others had been lost to miscarriage. According to her husband, she seemed to have experienced an episode of postpartum delirium after her second pregnancy but had no follow-up. During this most recent birth, emergency services took Mrs. Kouyate to the maternity ward, while Sadio was taken to an intensive care unit.

The referral letter the hospital team sent to Minkowska stated that Mrs. Kouyate displayed "an ill-adapted behavior and difficulties to establish a relation with her child, including a refusal to acknowledge the child's gender and first name." The hospital team added that the linguistic barrier and cultural differences "made her stay at the maternity ward complicated, but that she was able to express her refusal to breastfeed and not participate in any medical care." Meanwhile, Sadio was transferred to the neonatology unit for premature intensive care. With encouragement from the hospital's health-care teams and Mrs. Kouyate's family, the relationship between mother and child was progressively established. But persistent problems in the case included communication issues between Mr. and Mrs. Kouyate and a refusal by both to accept any outside assistance, including a referral to an ethnopsychiatrist.

The letter then described that "the mother's mental confusion, the divergence between the father['s] and the mother's version of events surrounding the birth of Sadio, and explorations as to whether any follow-up would be possible for the family, together motivate us to seek advice on how to understand Sadio's status and how to help the family." The referral included a separate letter from Mrs. Kouyate's social worker, who echoed the maternity professionals' concern and added that while Mrs. Kouyate was initially opposed to a meeting with Centre Minkowska, she had eventually accepted it "so that she could prove she was not sick in her head." Through exchanges with hospital professionals, Dr. Bennegadi gathered enough information to deduce that Mrs. Kouyate seemed to be experiencing delusions of persecution, with interpretive mechanisms suggesting paranoia, and that she identified Mr. Kouyate as her persecutor. Dr. Bennegadi called Mr. Kouyate to see if someone else from the family, whom Mrs. Kouyate trusted, could accompany her to the center. In the end, Mrs. Kouyate refused to come. Meanwhile, the social worker continued to voice her concern for the children in the Kouyate family and began to talk about reporting the situation (un signalement). All the Kouyate children showed learning and speech delays and, according to the social worker, displayed strange behavior. Mrs. Kouyate continued to be agitated, continually criticizing and threatening her husband, while the latter appeared attentive and concerned. In written correspondence with Centre Minkowska, I learned that the Center for Mother and Infant Protection (PMI) reported that Mrs. Kouyate came every week and complained about her husband. However, the family's appointed child psychiatrist appeared to believe that Mrs. Kouyate's behavioral disorders—her distanced behavior and lack of interactions with her children—had progressively disappeared and that she was taking good care of the children.

Two years later, in 2008, Centre Minkowska was contacted by the special educator of Child Protection Services (ASE, Aide sociale à l'enfance) for transcultural psychiatry support. Following a report by ASE and an audience with a judge, all the Kouyate children were placed in foster care, and parental visits were allowed under the condition that Mrs. Kouyate accept psychiatric care. Mrs. Kouyate did not attend the ruling and therefore had not heard the court-ordered treatment obligation. That same day, the juvenile squad picked up the children after school to place them in foster care. Mr. Kouyate called the center to inform us that his wife still refused to seek care. He asked for an appointment to discuss alternative solutions. During the meeting, after careful evaluation of the recent situation and acknowledgment of the concern raised by all professionals caring for the Kouyate family, Dr. Bennegadi decided that the only solution was to organize a type of involuntary hospitalization for Mrs. Kouyate at the request of a third party (*hospitalization à la demande d'un tiers*).

To do this, Mr. Kouyate and the children's psychiatrist had to write formal letters advocating for Mrs. Kouyate's hospitalization. Although Mrs. Kouyate opposed being taken to the hospital, she was not aggressive when it occurred. A week later, the hospital's psychiatrist, whom I will refer to as Dr. Duriez, contacted Dr. Bennegadi because she was at a loss about what to do regarding Mrs. Kouyate and sought a "more appropriate" structure that would share responsibility for therapy. She noted she was looking for a place where her patient's culture would be "understood." The family mediator had informed Dr. Duriez that Mr. Kouyate was planning to take his wife back to Mali to be cured. According to him, she refused to go out of fear that she would be unable to return to France and that her husband would instead take back a new, younger wife.

When we arrived on the scene, Marie-Jo, Salimata, and I had to traverse a series of locked doors to access the psychiatry ward. Its atmosphere was tense, and we encountered delirious and physically debilitated patients on our way to see Mrs. Kouyate. The ward, a public structure, was devoid of any aesthetic warmth. Its walls were either bare concrete or painted white. Staff at the ward directed us upstairs, where we met Mr. and Mrs. Kouyate, who were waiting for us. It was at this point that Marie-Jo realized that Mrs. Kouyate spoke Khasonke, not Soninke. It had been Minkowska's responsibility to call in a professional interpreter, but no one knew when or how the mistake relating to the language choice had happened. Unfortunately, Salimata did not speak Khasonke. This was a significant disappointment for Mr. Kouyate, who had been waiting weeks for this meeting—and for us. Mrs. Kouyate, on the other hand, appeared expressionless. Salimata said she could contact a friend by phone who could help, but we knew that doing so would undermine some of the reasons for this visit—to facilitate trust, easy interaction, and a solid foundation for the patient-doctor relationship between Mrs. Kouyate and Marie-Jo. As I watched the scene unfold, I wondered how Mrs. Kouyate might feel; she had been isolated in the ward for almost two months, removed from her children, and had no significant conversational partners or means to express herself. At the time, I thought the violence of this situation itself might drive a person to a state of madness.

Dr. Duriez arrived considerably late to our scheduled appointment. She greeted us all but seemed rushed and distracted. Marie-Jo introduced me as a visiting anthropologist doing research at the center. The psychiatrist firmly shook my hand and said, "Great! You speak African?" Disconcerted by her abruptness and the way she glossed all languages on the continent through the generic label "African," I did not have time to answer before she turned to Salimata and asked the same question. Marie-Jo pointed out to the psychiatrist that she had mistaken Mrs. Kouyate's language and that for today's meeting, we would have to resort to using a translator by phone. "It's not possible, it's not possible," the psychiatrist repeated. "This is a disaster. What are we going to do? *I* sure don't know what to do anymore! Do you realize how important this was going to be? How long I've been waiting for *your intervention?*" (emphasis in original). Exasperated, she rushed us all into a consultation room and asked a nurse and a psychology intern to join us. The eight of us crowded into the very small room, which had only a desk, a telephone, and enough chairs for us to sit.

The psychiatrist first asked Mr. Kouyate's permission to have the Minkowska team attend and intervene during the consultation, and then she asked him how Mrs. Kouyate was doing. Mr. Kouyate replied that ever since she had been hospitalized, things were much better. Now she actually answered when he greeted her. The psychiatrist turned to Mrs. Kouyate and asked whether she agreed. Mrs. Kouyate answered that she was not sick. Aggressively, the psychiatrist explained to Mrs. Kouyate that the French republic has laws and that if she refused treatment, her children would remain in foster care. Mr. Kouyate then translated her comments to his wife in Khasonke. Pointing to her back, Mrs. Kouyate responded that the only thing wrong with her is that she sometimes hurt "there." The psychiatrist turned to us, exasperated. As Mr. Kouyate was translating for his wife, the psychiatrist said, "See what difficulties I have to face? . . . [It is like] I am practicing veterinary medicine. I do admit that Mrs. Kouyate looks more relaxed, but she is delirious, and I cannot access her delirium. The major concern now is to get her to understand this law issue and the legal implications of her forced hospitalization. Someone must explain to her that I will not let her out unless she agrees to regularly go to a place [mental health consultation] where someone speaks African."

Turning to Marie-Jo, the psychiatrist asked whether the center was able to provide drug injections. Mr. Kouyate interrupted to say that his wife wanted to know why the state had taken her children. The psychiatrist ignored him and turned back to Marie-Jo, pursuing the subject of treatment: "She must have one injection per month." Marie-Jo replied that this type of service was not provided at Centre Minkowska. Meanwhile, after Mr. Kouyate translated what was being said, Mrs. Kouyate shook her head in a sign of refusal. Noticing this, the psychiatrist, increasingly agitated, replied, "But you *must!*" (emphasis in original).

At that point, to defuse the situation, Marie-Jo suggested that it might be better to get a Khasonke interpreter from Inter-Migrant Services (ISM).[1] Mr. Kouyate interjected to say that even if we called for an interpreter, his wife would not change her mind and would not listen to us. "She simply does not understand why the state has taken her children," he repeated. Through translation, he then reiterated to his wife the necessity for her to accept treatment involving a slow-release injection if she wanted to be released from the hospital and get her children back. Meanwhile, I asked the psychiatrist whether she had heard about ISM. She had, but she insisted that their services would not be enough; she needed help from professionals familiar with "African customs" or from "an African psychiatrist who can deal with Africans."

The psychiatrist then told Mrs. Kouyate that she would also have to go to consultations at Centre Minkowska, where there would be a translator. Trying to get a better grasp of the situation, Marie-Jo asked the psychiatrist what Mrs. Kouyate had said when she spoke of feeling unwell. "Does she talk about *djinns*, about *maraboutage*, about *seitan?*" she asked.

The psychiatrist turned to Mr. Kouyate: "You said that, before, you would bring rice bags to Mrs. Kouyate, and she thought they were poisoned." Before waiting for an answer, she picked up the phone, called ISM, and was connected to a Khasonke translator. She then addressed Mr. Kouyate again: "Mr. Kouyate, explain to the interpreter what the problem is—that she refused to feed her children, and that she didn't want to put food in the fridge." She passed the phone to Mr. Kouyate, who spoke with the interpreter. The psychiatrist, restless by this point, snatched the phone out of Mr. Kouyate's hands.

The translator, now on speakerphone, explained that according to Mr. Kouyate, his wife would not agree to go to external consultations. At home, she had refused to cook and feed her children, and she insulted Mr. Kouyate all night long. Even the children were afraid to approach her. He said that Mr. Kouyate felt angry because she always took the children away when he held them in his arms.

While Mrs. Kouyate responded to the interpreter, the psychiatrist said to us: "See, evidently there is also a conjugal problem which I can't access, either." The interpreter then translated Mrs. Kouyate's response for us:

> Mrs. Kouyate explains that her last child was born prematurely, and that she was placed in an infant foster care home shortly after she left the maternity clinic. According to her, the problem was that Mr. Kouyate refused to take care of the child. As far as she's concerned, Mrs. Kouyate never caused him financial problems. During her pregnancy, her husband asked her how she had gotten pregnant. She told him she had never been with anyone else. Still, Mr. Kouyate refused to take care of the child. Moreover, as their marriage was arranged between families, he went and told everyone she was crazy. She explains that she belongs to the griot caste, and therefore she sometimes sings the songs of her country. Because of that, Mr. Kouyate claims that she is crazy, when in fact, singing simply makes her feel happy.

The psychiatrist was surprised at the mention of Mr. Kouyate's questions around the child's paternity; she had never heard this concern before. "See, she has to be dealt with by Africans!" She then informed us that Mrs. Kouyate firmly contended in their discussions that her last child was not a girl but a boy named Sadio. The interpreter proceeded to translate this information to Mr. and Mrs. Kouyate. At that point, Mrs. Kouyate was able to rectify the misunderstanding: she never said that Sadio was not a girl. Rather, she said that she had lost twins before Sadio was born, and as Salimata explained, among the griot caste, after the death of twins, it is customary to name the following child Sadio, which is a gender-neutral name.

In response to this new information, the psychiatrist said, "See, I don't know these things. I'm drowning. How can I practice psychoanalysis under these conditions?" Turning to Marie-Jo, she asked, "Do you have psychiatrists who speak African?"

There then followed a series of exchanges during which Mrs. Kouyate voiced accusations related to her husband rejecting the children but also responded to her husband's own allegations, namely that she sometimes refused to feed the children. She explained that the children themselves did not always appreciate the food that Mr. Kouyate brought home, giving the example of her daughter Fatoumata, who once told her mother that the tubs of yogurt her father brought home were sometimes past the recommended date of consumption. "When did the problems start, then?" Dr. Duriez asked. Mrs. Kouyate responded by commenting on her husband's occasional violent behavior, referring to an episode in which she had to hide and the firemen had to intervene. Seeing Dr. Duriez's astonishment when listening to these unknown details, Salimata commented that professionals had only listened to Mr. Kouyate, and that this distorted everything.

MR. K: It's in 2002, after Fatoumata's birth [the second child], that the illness started. At that point, we had no problems. She's the one who is sick. Just take a look at the file written up by the judge for children. As far as I'm concerned, I have nothing to blame myself for.

DR. D: There are two things that are important at the moment, Mr. Kouyate. The first one is for me to be able to send your wife to a psychiatrist at Minkowska. The second is that this woman, whether she is sick or not, is in a context which I yet have to understand. But to put it bluntly, I'm fed up with this. I really need to obtain this permission to send her to Minkowska.

At that point, Marie-Jo asked Salimata whether she thought Mrs. Kouyate spoke coherently—a detail transcultural clinicians sometimes ask during interpreter-mediated sessions, to identify potential signs of psychosis. Salimata responded that she could not answer this question on the basis of a single phone interview. Shortly thereafter, Mrs. Kouyate asserted that she had no illness, that the cause of her behavior was due to her husband's doubt, and that what had triggered their problems was that he had said she was crazy and he was going to divorce her. At the time, she had told him that she would agree to a divorce but would not move—that she would stay in France, where he brought her in the first place.

For Dr. Duriez, it seemed as if further details held no weight at that point. Addressing Mrs. Kouyate directly, she reiterated that she would not discharge her from the hospital as long as she refused to see a doctor at Centre Minkowska.

Turning to Marie-Jo, she explained that she could not do her job unless she had more information about the context.

MR. K: She already knows the psychiatrist from Minkowska. I can already tell you, she won't agree to go.

DR. D: Really, we're in African times. . . . We are attending a three-way deaf conversation.

Marie-Jo then carefully tried to explain Centre Minkowska's clinical medical anthropology (AMC) framework to Dr. Duriez. The psychiatrist, exasperated, barely seemed to listen. She responded that she could no longer put up with such work conditions. She said she found no gratification in her work, spoke of "professional narcissism," and said that she could not do her job properly when overwhelmed. Marie-Jo attempted to explain that being an expert on "African culture" was not the key to unlocking the Kouyates' situation. She discussed the concept of explanatory models and the AMC framework's disease, illness, and sickness diagnostic triad. She then told the psychiatrist that the key to understanding a case like the Kouyates' was for the mental health practitioner to respectfully accept and consider the patient's illness representations; in turn, the patient would be more likely to be open to receiving the practitioner's advice about treatment. Leaning over the desk, holding her head in her hands, the psychiatrist appeared to be utterly burned out professionally. Sighing deeply, she simply reiterated her unhelpful working conditions, dismissing Marie-Jo's comments. We left after Marie-Jo agreed to schedule an appointment at Centre Minkowska with Dr. Sarr and a Khasonke interpreter, on the condition that Mrs. Kouyate would agree to the extended-release drug regimen and a meeting with the Minkowska team. Marie-Jo then scheduled the appointment with Mr. Kouyate on the basis that his wife would eventually accept the psychiatrist's treatment and be allowed out of the hospital.

On our way back to Centre Minkowska, Marie-Jo and Salimata heatedly discussed the psychiatrist's attitude. They described her as infantilizing the Kouyates and addressing them in a way she would never address white French patients. They were shocked at her use of the expression "veterinary medicine" at the beginning of the conversation. "She may suffer from professional burn-out," Marie-Jo commented, "but that is no excuse to treat her patient the way she does." They lamented Mrs. Kouyate's fate and affirmed the necessity of finding a way to have her attend a consultation on her own, without her husband, so that she might feel less defensive. Marie-Jo also commented that the danger with MEDIACOR is that it can be used by some referring agents, such as this psychiatrist, as an easy answer for their unwillingness to treat some migrant patients or as an exit door to escape the complexity of certain situations.

On the day of the appointment, Mr. and Mrs. Kouyate both arrived at Centre Minkowska. Mrs. Kouyate had eventually agreed to the drug regimen; her children, however, were still in foster care. Unfortunately, because ISM failed to respond to Centre Minkowska's request for a Khasonke translator, Dr. Bennegadi was forced to reschedule the appointment, re-contact ISM, and send the couple back home. At the second appointment, Dr. Bennegadi gathered Mr. and Mrs. Kouyate, the Khasonke translator, Marie-Jo, a secretary, and me in the mediation room. The goal of that meeting, Dr. Bennegadi later explained to me, was to reassure Mrs. Kouyate that Centre Minkowska held a different position than the hospital's psychiatrist, which he hoped would make her feel less defensive and more open to therapy. With Mr. Kouyate, Dr. Bennegadi also intended to broach the possibility of one-on-one therapy sessions as a way to show respect for his position as the family decision-maker. Although I left France shortly after, Marie-Jo informed me that Mrs. Kouyate had maintained her drug regimen and was receiving therapy at her district's CMP with a different psychiatrist.

A SUCCESSFUL INTERVENTION?

This MEDIACOR intervention in this case could be considered successful in at least one important way: Mrs. Kouyate's state of health improved. Also, through the intervention of staff at Centre Minkowska, she was extricated from the psychiatric ward—an environment in which she was being mistreated by her appointed mental health practitioner and which could have further damaged her mental health. Mrs. Kouyate's children remained in foster care; the judge on her case considered her recovery too recent and her stabilization still precarious. However, because of her progress, the judge allowed parental visits on Sundays. Despite these markers of success, I consider the overall context of therapy I witnessed utterly dehumanizing.

My impression is influenced particularly by the hospital psychiatrist's references to practicing what she called "veterinary medicine" and the infantilizing way she addressed the Kouyates. The psychiatrist's method for dealing with her patient's cultural difference involved a combination of ignorance (e.g., her belief that a single "African language" exists) and stigmatizing comments about a kind of generic African "other" (e.g., "She has to be dealt with by Africans" and "We're in African times"). As I witnessed the exchanges, I was reminded of Frantz Fanon's (1973) description of the conditions in which those labeled "mentally ill" were treated in colonial Algeria. The violence of the situation, which lay in the health-care professional's dehumanization of her patient and racist essentialization, is reminiscent of French colonial psychiatrists' attitudes toward African colonial subjects. Some scholars, such as Italian psychiatrist and anthropologist Roberto Beneduce (2016), have described how the mental health symptoms experienced by various African migrants are related to their own life trajectories and events but also reminiscent of a collective, traumatic colonial past. Through this vignette, we see how the legacy of the colonial psychiatry paradigm can manifest through the practices of current psychiatry professionals—to the extent that encounters with foreigners, such as North and sub-Saharan Africans, represent the contemporary epitome of otherness in the French context. Professionals like Dr. Duriez feel as though they require expert knowledge and have no way of relating to such patients. While her attitude should not be generalized to represent how all referring institutional actors handle migrants, her overall attitude about feeling unable *from the onset* to address migrant patients' needs *because* of their cultural difference is a pattern I have seen among institutional actors from all sectors. It is also a pattern widely acknowledged by specialized mental health centers. The very existence of MEDIACOR attests to that.

At a deeper level, this case attests to how colonization has irreparably transformed the gaze of modern democracies to the point that violence and subjugation are legitimized through contemporary mental health practice (Mbembe 2016). There is a double violence to the Kouyates' situation. Through the psychiatrists' comments, Mrs. Kouyate is reduced to an object deprived of any ability to express herself. In this context, her two major mediators simultaneously act as persecutors: her husband—her designated interpreter—and the psychiatrist—the embodiment of the state that took her children away. As a translator, on the one hand, Mr. Kouyate had control over his wife's narrative and probably had an interest in not engaging with his own responsibility for his wife's distress. The psychiatrist, on the other hand, did not have the necessary distance or willingness to get around the linguistic obstacle other than relying on Mr. Kouyate as an interpreter. And what can be said of Centre Minkowska's response to this case? Marie-Jo's attempt to mitigate the hospital psychiatrist's comments about her inability to treat Mrs. Kouyate, as well as to sensitize her to an alternative perspective on the doctor-patient relationship, categorically failed. In some respects, Marie-Jo even appeared to legitimize the psychiatrist's culturalist interpretation of Mrs. Kouyate's case through justifying her presence at the hospital and positioning herself as a cultural expert. This can be seen when Marie-Jo asks the psychiatrist whether Mrs. Kouyate talks about "*djinns*, about *maraboutage*, about *seitan*?"

Ultimately, by agreeing to receive Mrs. Kouyate at the center, and thus to be perceived as a place where African doctors can deal with African people, Marie-Jo acted as a representative of Centre Minkowska and indirectly legitimized a regulative system at the margins of which it operates as an institutional dead end. By "regulative system," I refer to the fact that state institutions police individuals, and that migrants—designated as problematic and undesirable populations—are under particular scrutiny (Fassin et al. 2013). In this case, the work of state agents, beyond their explicit mission of caring for and accompanying the Kouyate family, may also produce abusive and stigmatizing situations as they attempt to have the Kouyates "fit in" with the system—to speak French, adapt to local norms of parent-child bonding, and so on. In this situation, no less than ten state agents were involved: a family mediator, a hospital psychiatrist, a hospital care team, a social worker, a child psychiatrist, a special educator at ASE, a juvenile squad, foster care services, a PMI team, and a judge. As the "regulating" still proved ineffective, cultural expertise as provided by Centre Minkowska was called on to respond to the powerlessness of state agents and provide intelligibility to a situation otherwise interpreted as dysfunctional. This is one example of the double bind in which staff at specialized mental health centers often find themselves: they contest the stigmatization of their migrant patients while legitimizing it through positioning themselves—and being identified by others—as "cultural" experts. Although Mrs. Kouyate was successfully reintegrated into a mainstream public health structure thanks to Minkowska's intervention, the challenge of this stigmatizing referral is only met halfway. In the end, Centre Minkowska had little if no impact on the structural determinants that continued to weigh on this family. The success, if any, resided in the center's ability to mediate between state institutions (over three years, in this case) and give consideration to the multiple levels of complexity (individual, institutional, societal) that this case presented, in order to find a solution that avoided further stigmatization.

THE UNDERLYING DYNAMICS OF DISCRIMINATION

The concept of discrimination is central to understanding the dynamics of the Kouyates' experience. While her treatment of the Kouyate couple seemed extremely dehumanizing and infantilizing, Dr. Duriez seemed completely unaware of her own biases as she tried to provide care. My research methodology did not allow me to interrogate Dr. Duriez about her reasons for treating the Kouyates the way she did, and the sociopolitical context in France makes it challenging for scholars to write about or even research the topic. As French anthropologists Chantal Crenn and Laurence Kotobi (2012) have illustrated in an edited volume on ethnicity in France, the "ethnicisation" of social relations in French society, and the anxiety it has generated, has had an impact on the ways that French researchers relate to their subjects. As a result, the concept of ethnicity had long been absent in French academia and reemerged almost inadvertently in studies on immigration (De Rudder 1999). This lack of focus on ethnicity reflects France's construction as a nation-state founded on cultural unity, a common language, and a common history. The lack has also meant that other interpretations of immigration, such as Marxist notions on the economic exploitation of migrants, have long been privileged over attention to the hierarchical structure of French society along ethnic lines (Réa and Tripier 2008).

Today, a substantial body of research documents the complex economic difficulties confronted by North and sub-Saharan African migrants (and their descendants), including in relation to access to housing (Barou 1999; Pan Ké Shon and Scodellaro 2015; Péchu 1999; Rezkallah 2000; Simon 2003), educational segregation (Durpaire 2006; Ichou 2013), police profiling (Goris, Jobard, and Lévy 2009), discrimination in access to employment (Brinbaum, Meurs, and Primon 2015; Cediey and Foroni 2008), and high unemployment rates (Meurs, Pailhé, and Simon 2006; Silberman, Alba, and Fournier 2007). In industrial and service sectors, sub-Saharan African migrants were (and are) discriminated against in job training, promotion, and bonuses. Many are segregated in suburban high-rise housing projects on the basis of their African origin (Quiminal and Timera 2002, 23), and a recent report from the National Board of Media (CSA 2014) observed that "non-white" persons were more frequently discussed in negative terms (e.g., delinquents) than positive ones (e.g., business founders) within news reports.

Didier Fassin and colleagues in the fields of anthropology and sociology pioneered investigations into inequalities and discrimination in health in France (see Carde et al. 2002).[2] As they documented—and as Dr. Duriez's behavior illustrates—culture has been used as a determinant by all professionals who face problems in transcultural situations. This "reification" and "overdetermination" of culture to explain health differentials, French sociologist Marguerite Cognet (2007, 54) writes, conceals a number of social stakes: namely, it makes migrants responsible for their so-called ill-adapted behavior, avoids questioning the established social order, and absolves society of responsibility for social and economic inequalities. Beyond removing professionals of any responsibility in the face of potential misdiagnoses or other errors, this protracted focus on culture in health care avoids questioning the very relevance of public health interventions; it also justifies potentially ethically problematic practices, such as hospitalization under constraint and child placement, as in the Kouyates' case.

Dr. Duriez's reaction to the Kouyates also illustrates how France's immigration policies and political discourse around sub-Saharan African families have resulted in stigmatizing, generic definitions of "African" culture as pathological. Various studies conducted in France have established how biomedical institutions have perceived "cultural" dilemmas among their sub-Saharan African patients in the domains of infectious disease (Gilloire 2000; Kotobi 2000) and reproductive health (Sargent 2005; Sauvegrain 2012) in particular. In each case, essentializing depictions of culture have been used to characterize sub-Saharan Africans as a risk population, a rapidly growing population, and a population maladapted to its new environment. Against the national background of republican universalism and its related philosophy of health-care access for all, such cultural stigmatization for pragmatic reasons is unacknowledged.

It would be wrong to assume that concerns with the relevance of "culture" in care were necessarily underscored by discriminatory, regulating logics. For numerous institutional actors, it became clear that culturally diverse understandings of care and of other services accessed by migrants required culturally sensitive forms of intervention, such as that by trained interpreters, who could translate not only language but also ideas. Such intervention was paramount to improving patient care and interactions between migrant families and public institutions.

THE LANGUAGE OF WRITTEN REFERRALS: REPERTOIRES OF REPRESENTATIONS AND IDEOLOGY

Another way discrimination is built into referral encounters is through the language of the referral letter, not only in spoken discourse among professionals, as shown in the Kouyate vignette. I base my analysis on a sample of files of sub-Saharan African patients I had access to at Centre Minkowska and focus on their referral documents. Such documents are heterogeneous in form and origin, from handwritten individual requests for consultation to letter-headed court orders for therapy; combined, they illustrate the depth and breadth of state population management processes in the field of mental health. In a sample of ten referrals containing supplemental information, two came from the national education system (one from a school psychologist and the other from a school teacher), three from medical workers (two clinical psychologists and a pediatrician), two from social services, and three from legal services (one from a court order, one from a voluntary association in support of a court order, and one from child protection services). Most state institutions are thus represented in the sample. Documentation supplementing each referral varies, from inspired narratives on the patient's social history, to a school's student competence and knowledge evaluation, to a "social report" displaying the patient's family administrative status and financial details.

The expressed motivations for many of these referrals were couched in ambiguous terms related to "difficulties," "suffering," or "fragility." The exceptions were the referral from the pediatrician, who specified his patient's medical disorders ("relationship" and "invasive development" disorders) as the reason for referral, and the referral from the clinical psychologist, who directly referenced her patient's "depression, weight loss, and cannabis consumption" as a motive for referral. I draw attention here to the ambiguous ways patients' mental health is described prior to formal consultations with a psychiatrist; after all, such referrals may seek specialized mental health centers specifically to clarify a diagnosis. It becomes revealing, however, when considering how *unambiguously* referring institutional actors characterize relationships between patients' social history and cultural background. For instance, a link may be drawn between delinquency and culturally specific family arrangements, such as polygamy. The wording of such characterizations varies from one referral to another, and in some files, this connection is only made implicitly. Over the course of my research, I identified two major representation schemes common among referrals, which I detail in the next section. I draw attention to linguistic elements used to describe patients' social history, and I argue that these referrals rely heavily on a common (French) frame of semiotic reference to signal to readers that these migrant patients stand outside normal—mentally healthy—boundaries.

COMMUNICATING CULTURAL DIFFERENCES, LOCATING PATHOLOGY

Throughout this set of referral documents, I found references to patients' social history to be framed in terms of social precarity, "unusual" family arrangements, or both. Some referral letters included class-based forms of judgments that pathologized *banlieue* (suburb) lifestyles. For example, a middle school teacher wrote a request for a specialized mental health consultation and reported that she "noticed a singular form of suffering" in one of her students. The history she provided specified that the student resided in a "sensitive neighborhood and a *communautaire* (community-based, i.e.[,] ethnic-conflict prone) environment" and that his mother took trips to Mali without him. She noted child protection services had sent the student to a social shelter during one of these trips, and she hinted that his "singular form of suffering" might be related to his cultural origin and precarious social milieu.

Whether people realize it or not, their ideas about the *banlieue* lifestyle are often influenced by popular media. This holds particularly true for people who have never resided or spent much time in such an area. Life in the *banlieue* is commonly portrayed in the media through images of social precarity and delinquent youth—rough-looking young men in sportswear hanging out outside housing projects, images of dysfunctional households—characterized, for instance, by polygamy and large families crammed in small, deteriorating suburban apartments. All elements may be seen in the letter of a social worker discussing the case of a "juvenile delinquent." In it, the social worker narrated the youth's history, which included his delinquent acts (mainly theft), problems at school, and "fragility in the relationships he has and the choices he makes. . . . He has trouble saying 'no' to his entourage and asserting himself." In the referral, the social worker assumed the young man's actions and apparent difficulties communicating with his mother—with reference to him belonging to a female-headed household—were linked to his "communication difficulties" in general. Referrals are often thin in details. This thinness of details is significant, as referrals like this one generally failed to provide a complete picture of persons or nuances in describing their troubles. This letter presented the young man in a flat, one-dimensional, judgmental way.

Although one would expect referral letters to places like Centre Minkowska to emphasize mental suffering, in this sample I found several that seemed to focus primarily on referrers' perceptions of how patients' behavior and practices seemed culturally different. This was often coded linguistically through discourse about unusual family arrangements. Consider a letter from a social worker referring a separated Malian mother of four to Centre Minkowska. It first notes that the mother seems to have difficulties establishing a relationship with her fourth child, who was born "out-of-wedlock." The social worker then talks about what she perceives to be the patient's culturally distinct behavior: "She could not divorce because of family pressures." "She rarely looks at her child and calls her 'it.'" "She plans on entrusting her [the daughter] with her sister who lives in Mali and who does not have any children."[3] Only then, toward the end of the letter, does the social worker emphasize the patient's mental and physical distress: "She [the patient] says things like, 'If I keep thinking too much, my head will break' or 'my head spun and spun, and then it fell.'"

In another referral to the center, a clinical psychologist strongly emphasized the social precarity of his patient and appeared to identify his mixed cultural background as the root of his mental suffering. The clinical psychologist, who worked for a district's Department for Social Insertion, Fight against Exclusion and for Employment, wrote of a young unemployed man "in a state of deep suffering. Born in France, he lives between two cultures, which prevents him from establishing real identity markers (repères)." This comment reflects the state ideology's uneasiness with the concept of hybridity: in the Manichean opposition between the "immigré" and French categories, there seems to be no room for that concept (Taguieff [1987] 2001, 213).[4] Professionals at Centre Minkowska often commented on how France forces a cleavage of identities on migrants' descendants, resulting in mental suffering. In parentheses, the psychologist juxtaposed this diagnosis with a note that the young man's father had two wives and that he was raised by the second one. Implicitly, his notes presented the young man's family life as nonnormative, culturally specific, pathological, or, at the very least, worthy of particular attention. At the end of his letter, the psychologist gave his diagnosis of the patient: depression, weight loss, and cannabis consumption. He then juxtaposed this diagnosis with the patient's own interpretation of his suffering: "He believes to have been cursed (marabouté)."

In France, I would argue that the kind of vague language these state agents use stands for coded signs that are locally intelligible. For example, in another referral letter by a different clinical psychologist, who was caring for a woman and her four-year-old son's speech disabilities, the psychologist established the "*difficulties* experienced by Mrs. D. to *situate herself in her own history*. We thus thought of your consultation as *appropriate to her problem*, and we thought it would allow her to have support *from where she is situated*" (emphases mine). This last example aptly illustrates the art of coding cultural difference without naming it. Also, by referring the patient's mother to the center, this psychologist clearly though implicitly drew a relationship between the patient's already established disorder (speech impairment) and the parent's cultural difference (and related suffering). While it is reasonable to think a child may be affected by his parents' mental suffering, whether it stems from the experience of migrating or not, why is this connection left unarticulated in what is otherwise a very detailed referral letter? How does the language of referrals inscribe stigma on migrants, and what kind of stigma are referring agents perpetuating? Where do referring agents place blame for patients' suffering, and where do they locate the locus for change?

MANAGING MIGRANT FAMILIES

Such connections are partly influenced by common cultural representations of immigrants that stigmatize them on the grounds of social milieu and lifestyle. Indirectly, referring agents reproduce and disseminate these stereotypes. However, I suggest that the assumptions drawn about the risks immigrant patients incur from their social milieu and from their own social practices *also* imply that addressing a patient's "suffering" requires broader action by his or her entourage.

A pediatrician, the director of the Center for Early Medical and Social Action outside the Paris region, referred the mother of his four-year-old patient to the center "so that [she] can, in her language of origin, provide explanations on her son's *difficulties*" (emphasis mine). The child, the pediatrician indicated, suffered from "difficulties interacting" (*trouble relationnel*), exacerbated by "a pervasive developmental disorder." In the latest edition of the *Diagnostic and Statistical Manual of Mental Disorders*, this diagnosis has now been replaced with "autism spectrum disorders," a broad category that refers to various disorders characterized by delays in the development of basic functions such as communication and socialization. The doctor's report was accompanied by a handwritten letter from the child's father, who wondered whether his son was autistic and whether the doctor could provide medication to help his son sleep. He specified that his son's condition seemed to have been triggered by an episode of high fever when he was an infant. This letter led me to presume that the child's parents proposed a biomedical diagnosis that coincided with the pediatrician's. It also left me to ponder exactly why the pediatrician felt it necessary to refer the mother to a specialized mental health center: What other diagnosis might the mother offer that could facilitate this pediatrician's treatment of his patient? Nothing in the referral indicated that the mother was suffering from her son's situation—although she very well could be—or that she had requested psychological support from a place where she could easily express her distress (i.e., in her first language). Neither did the letter of referral establish that the mother had a different cultural explanation for her son's disorder that prevented her from accepting the situation or that explained her own distress. In the end, the pediatrician did not assume responsibility for treating the patient and placed the burden on the patient's mother. This case illustrates how the referring professional expected Minkowska staff to establish all these connections from common cultural coding strategies and collective representations.

Similarly, a Parisian court, ruling on two "juvenile delinquents" to be placed under an "educational assistance measure," ordered the delinquents' parents to go to a specialized mental health center. In the letter, the judge indicated that "a

consultation measure is entrusted to an ethnopsychiatry center [no specific institution is targeted] to allow Mr. and Mrs. D. to speak to therapists of their language and culture." The letter was accompanied in the patients' file with a copy of
the ruling, which added that "it is expected that light will be shed so that we can
apprehend the situation with respect to the cultural representations of [the] persons concerned. [This is] why we call for *an ethnoclinical intervention* of several
consultations (four maximum)" (emphasis mine). The letter specified that a report
was expected from the ethnopsychiatrist/ethnoclinician, and that consultation
fees would be paid for by the public treasury. No information was provided on
what may have led the judge to think there was any relationship between the
behavior of these two young "delinquents" and their parents' cultural representations. Did the judge see the young men's cultural ways (or their parents') as deviant, or did he or she suspect that their family environment was maladapted because
of culturally problematic child-rearing practices?

In these two cases, the relationship between cultural difference and mental
health suffering was unfounded. However, both referrals could be seen as attempts
on the part of the pediatrician and the judge to offer support services to populations that would otherwise be ignored in the first case or criminalized in the second. In both cases, the center's "cultural expertise," however it was perceived, not
only reached beyond mental health issues per se but served as a tool to manage
institutional dead ends. In other words, it may be that the referring agents did not
know how to help, communicate with, or handle the patients effectively, so they
shipped them off to the center. They may not have known what else to do—or
did not want to invest time trying to figure that out. They may even have considered places like Minkowska the "default" place for migrants to go for help. Regardless of their motivations, through the actions of referring agents the center
became a last-ditch place to send patients whose cases were considered too difficult for any mainstream service to handle. A pre-consultation meeting I attended
at Minkowska with Marie-Jo clearly illustrated this point.

Marie-Jo had met a psychologist working at a municipal career and support
center for youth in a northwestern suburb of Paris. The psychologist had contacted
Marie-Jo over the phone and expressed a desire to meet with her to discuss the
case of a twenty-two-year-old man she hoped to refer to the center. Marie-Jo
invited me to attend the meeting and introduced me as an anthropologist and affiliated researcher with the center. After the three of us sat down, Marie-Jo invited
the psychologist, Mrs. Pierre, to tell us about this young man, named Idriss, whom
she had assisted at the career center. Mrs. Pierre started by specifying that Idriss
was French born and that she was unsure whether he was of Malian or Senegalese origin. From what Idriss told her, he had been taken "home" (*au pays*) by his
father when he was five and had come back to France when he was nineteen years
old. His mother had passed away, but Mrs. Pierre did not know when. Idriss had
a stutter. He had never gone to school, either "at home" or in France, because his

maternal grandfather did not want him to. "What about the Quranic school?" Marie-Jo interjected. Mrs. Pierre thought he had not gone to Quranic school, either, but she was not sure. She had been informed, however, that he was the only one among his siblings not to have been sent to school. When Marie-Jo asked her what Idriss's position among his siblings was, Mrs. Pierre was again unable to answer.

Mrs. Pierre then informed us that when Idriss came back to France, his father stayed "home." Idriss thus came to stay with "a lady" he called his aunt, apparently his father's second wife, with whom he did not get along. "I suspect she beats him. I don't have proof of that, but I do know for sure that she rejects him, and that they have an extremely difficult relationship," Mrs. Pierre said. Idriss's main problem, she explained, was that he could neither read nor write. His stutter added to these handicaps and made it difficult for him to find a job. He had been hired by a state-sponsored association that assisted unqualified youth to find a job. Thanks to this program, he had been working on a construction site, where he was being trained as a heavy machinery operator. He had already failed the qualifying test once, but his employers were still "very satisfied" with his work. They found him to be "responsible, reliable, and amiable." They worked hard to find him a real job before his contract with the association ended. "But there's another problem," Mrs. Pierre added, "which is about his supplemental health coverage (*mutuelle*). He pays for it, but his father manages it 'from home.' So, when Idriss gets reimbursed from his health care expenses, his dad is the one collecting the money." She explained that Idriss needed to obtain a separate bank account. He had been assisted by the career and support center's social workers to take measures that would help him open the account, but Idriss's aunt had refused to provide them with a housing certificate. Mrs. Pierre recounted that this prompted her to call the aunt herself, but since "the aunt expressed herself very badly," she sought the help of a French-speaking family member and managed to obtain the certificate. Unfortunately, one piece of documentation was still missing, which was the copy of the aunt's residency permit.

Mrs. Pierre returned to Idriss's stuttering problem. She explained that he had been going to a speech therapist for about three months, and that this had enabled him to progress rapidly. But because of the health coverage issue, he had been unable to pursue therapy. "Paradoxically," Mrs. Pierre added, "the progress he made expressing himself better has enabled him to socialize with people more easily, which led him to hang out with the youth in his neighborhood. Not a good thing, these boys. They are all involved in small delinquency and theft. I'm concerned Idriss will go down the same path." She then complained about how people who are supposed to assist Idriss at the youth center had a bad attitude. "Especially the district's social worker, who keeps repeating there is nothing she can do for Idriss, even though she has always been unwilling to even call his aunt." Mrs. Pierre proceeded to talk about herself and how she felt overwhelmed at work, helpless in her attempt to have work colleagues collaborate with one another and, in this case, with Idriss's family. She was the only one to have gone to the trouble of contacting the family, whom she found "very nice and available." She was, however, limited by precarious work conditions at the youth center; her contract was renewed every three months, and she worked only four hours a week. "I'll tell you, this doesn't make one feel like investing oneself in the job. We can't possibly do everything. We're not gods!"

Finally, Mrs. Pierre asked Marie-Jo how Centre Minkowska could help her. "What cultural aspects would help me better understand Idriss's situation?" She suddenly turned to me: "What if he were a child-sorcerer, what would that mean? How would things go?" Seeing my puzzlement at the bluntness of the question and its awkward content, Marie-Jo jumped in to suggest various scenarios in which Idriss's specific position among his siblings and the conditions of his childhood might have affected his relationship with his family, specifically with his father. "But all of these are hypotheses, considering I don't have enough information to guide me here," Marie-Jo said. Nonetheless Mrs. Pierre returned to those scenarios, only to ask again how such cultural clues would help clarify Idriss's situation. Marie-Jo noted, "Well, at this point, I'm afraid I don't have much to offer in terms of explanation. I could offer to contact and meet with the aunt. I could also contact the district's social worker." Mrs. Pierre rolled her eyes. Marie-Jo continued, "Once contact has been made with the family, a mediation could take place." Mrs. Pierre responded that the priority now was to help Idriss become independent in terms of health-care coverage and housing. In response, Marie-Jo cautioned her not to destabilize family relations. She offered to be available by phone if Mrs. Pierre needed further assistance. She then launched into her presentation of the AMC approach. I asked Mrs. Pierre where she had heard about Centre Minkowska. She said that she had indirectly heard about the center when she was taking psychology classes at the university and was learning about ethnopsychiatry.

In this case, although Idriss's psychologist, Mrs. Pierre, talked about relevant factors in Idriss's case, she also commented on obstacles that are less psychological and more structural in nature. Idriss's family history indirectly produced a complicated administrative situation, which the psychologist was having trouble resolving, partly because of language obstacles; she referenced Idriss's aunt's speaking abilities. Idriss's lack of schooling further complicated his already precarious situation and seriously limited his opportunities for financial independence and social autonomy more generally. There were also stigmatizing assumptions in the psychologist's narrative, such as her characterization of Idriss's family structure as deviant ("a lady" he calls his aunt), which emphasized cultural issues over class-related ones. Other examples include her references to a violent suburban environment: "I suspect she beats him." "The youth in his neighborhood . . . they are all involved in small delinquency and theft."

This ambivalence, between acknowledging concrete structural inequalities and making sense of them as ineluctably linked to representations of what migrant life and lifestyles were like, was often expressed in such pre-consultation meetings with institutional actors. Frequently accompanying these narratives were expressions of professional burnout and feelings of discouragement at having to face such complicated situations. Cases involving migrants and their descendants were thus often portrayed by referring agents as "difficult" to deal with and as institutional dead ends.

How, then, do these agents come to a decision to refer patients to a place like Centre Minkowska? The psychologist's request was for Marie-Jo to elucidate a structural conundrum—not a mental health issue. Her insistent demands for Marie-Jo to provide a cultural analysis of the situation eventually led Marie-Jo to position herself as a cultural expert, even though she did so with great reluctance: "All of these are hypotheses." In this vignette, Mrs. Pierre, the referring state agent, demonstrated anxieties that were both personal—she goes out of her way to assist Idriss—and social, related to broader, overlapping cultural representations and structural constraints. "Culture" was thus used as a ready-made script to elucidate highly complex situations from which everyone was tempted to disengage.

INTERPRETERS AND THE "LANGUAGE BARRIER"

TEF: So, this person is referred to us by the Center where he is housed. They [referring professionals] tried to set up interviews with him, but they couldn't because of the language barrier.

DR. B: We don't use that kind of expression [language barrier] at Minkowska!

TEF: Well, that's what's written here!

DR. B: Well, you don't have to repeat their mistake! (*Laughs.*) Can a language ever become a barrier? Never! Who is facing the barrier? Not the person herself! The language is never a barrier. It's a linguistic issue (*une problématique linguistique*).

One aspect of France's uneasy relationship with its population's multiculturalism is the lack of national policy around interpreter services in public institutions. It was only in 2017 that a law intended to modernize the French health-care system was passed, which included an article on the importance of interpreters and health mediators to ensure health-care access to vulnerable populations. Prior to this, the interpreter profession in France had developed informally and often within associations created by migrants themselves. Even now, there are no national standards or certification for interpreters in French public services. There are budgets allocated to health structures for professional interpreter services, but health-care professionals are rarely informed of these funds or trained to work with interpreters. As a result, many rely on informal interpreters—bilingual colleagues or family and community members (Kotobi, Larchanché, and Kessar 2013).

Three-quarters of referrals directed to Centre Minkowska are based on the notion of a linguistic barrier. While Centre Minkowska was founded on the idea that patients would be able to elaborate their trauma or distress more clearly if speaking in their first languages, historical diversification in immigration flows has resulted in the fact that direct linguistic matches are often not possible. Recent arrivals of asylum seekers from countries like Afghanistan, Pakistan, Sudan, or Eritrea have increased the need for languages most clinicians cannot speak. The center has had to rely increasingly on professional linguistic interpreters, but the budget for such expenses has remained stable for years.

The overall budget from the Regional Health Agency has decreased yearly, disproportionately affecting health institutions that rent building space in Paris, as Centre Minkowska does (rental rates comprise a large part of overall budgets). To fund interpreter services, health institutions such as hospitals and CMPs have access to a specific budget dedicated to facilitate health-care access for "precarious populations" (known as *MIG Précarité*). This budget amount is calculated for each institution depending on the estimated proportion of precarious patients to whom they cater. This budget is not specifically dedicated to interpreting costs and must be balanced with other expenses. The budget proportion dedicated to interpreter services will thus vary from one institution to another. This funding is not available to social service institutions, such as Centers for Asylum Seekers (CADA, les Centres d'accueil pour demandeurs d'asile) or ASE—both of which also regularly refer patients to Centre Minkowska for linguistic reasons.

This context has become a major point of tension for clinicians now faced with budget shortages. In January 2017, Marie-Jo organized a meeting at the center to discuss the issue and invited the general director, Christophe Paris, and the psychiatrists. As head of MEDIACOR, Marie-Jo often found herself caught between the stark rise in referrals that required interpreters and the director's warning that she must limit interpreter services due to budget constraints. Dr. Cheref, who regularly works with Marie-Jo to evaluate patients' demands in the context of MEDIACOR, complained that it had become unbearable for him to receive those patients; he knew very well that he would be unable to offer them proper follow-up without access to an interpreter. As he explained, "How can I work under such conditions? I would rather not see the patients at all. If I see someone in really bad shape, or suicidal, in need of a medical treatment, and I am unable to follow up, what decision do I make? How do I do my job?" Dr. Cheref raised critical ethical questions with which we were familiar at the center, and we were often surprised that referring institutional actors did not ask themselves these questions when assisting non-francophone migrants. Dr. Cheref revealed that the logics of triage inherent to MEDIACOR's process of referral are tested when staff members meet a person during an evaluation: How do you let that person go, for economic reasons, when the encounter reinforces your sense of responsibility and engagement?

For Dr. Bennegadi, who also attended the meeting, the question need not even be asked—the answer is clear, since it invokes clinicians' foundational ethics. In response to Dr. Cheref, Dr. Bennegadi firmly said, "As a psychiatrist, I must attend to the person first and foremost. The cost of the interpreter for the institution is not my problem. This [treating patients] is our mission, and the institution needs to take the necessary actions in order to solve budget issues." Those of us who gathered debated this critical issue, which affected everyday practice, and discussed questions around the ethics of clinicians in the face of the managerial logics of health care and related budget cuts. Through the elaboration of their positions, we see a contradiction between Dr. Cheref's everyday ethics, calibrated to his near-at-hand experience in undertaken patient evaluations, and Dr. Bennegadi's reference to normative ethics about beneficence that, in his viewpoint, should be applied universally. While the universal ethical ideal of beneficence is one that all staff at Centre Minkowska support, the reality is that it is deeply challenged by on-the-ground practice. In that respect, even Dr. Bennegadi must be more nuanced when he negotiates those realities.

The following MEDIACOR situation illustrates these ethical dynamics in practice. A twenty-five-year-old Tamil-speaking man from Sri Lanka, who arrived in France in 2017 after fleeing from political persecution, was being housed in a CADA with his wife and daughter. Shortly after arriving in France, he suffered a stroke and was hospitalized. During his stay, he was diagnosed with a neurodegenerative disease. The referral to Centre Minkowska, written by the CADA's social worker, made no mention of whether this man had been able to speak with an interpreter. According to her, he was not clear at all about what his ailment entailed. He was extremely anxious, though, because his father died from a disease that had never been formally diagnosed, and he was afraid he was doomed with the same affliction. He was also very stressed because of his administrative situation.

DR. B: (*Interrupting the case presentation.*) But why? Why did she [the social worker] think of us? For god sake! That's just terrible!

MJ: It's because of the language!

DR. B: The language issue? I mean, he was seen at [Parisian hospital of high repute]. They could have very well set up a social and psychological follow-up for him! So that's exactly what we are going to recommend. Please write up a response stating that, in the follow-up service, which probably resorts to an interpreter at some point (*Marie-Jo snorts in disbelief*), we recommend that they organize for psychological support, as well. I mean, what is it about dispersing people in different directions, following a "Go there, they speak your language" type of rationale? It makes no sense!

MJ: So we tell them to refer the patient to the psychologist back at [Parisian hospital of high repute]?

DR. B: Ask them that the follow-up [at that hospital] be facilitated by an interpreter, which they likely already resorted to . . . I mean, hopefully! And if they haven't, then that's a way of saying, "Do it!" in a quite elegant manner. And then let's wait and see what they answer. If they refuse . . . I mean, I highly doubt it, I know the neurology team there, I would really be surprised. But if they answer negatively, you negotiate peacefully, you negotiate by saying that the ideal would be for an on-site psychologist to see him. They should have one within their unit. The problem is the interpreter. You have to explain it to them. . . . If they respond they have no interpreter, don't tell them "Well how did you know to explain the disease to him?" and vex them. You tell them, "It is very easy to call Inter-Service Migrants and rely on them to ensure the connection between neurological follow-up and psychological follow-up," and then we'll see. I mean, that's the least that can be done. His disease is serious enough so that someone [should] make efforts to call for an interpreter and explain things to him properly! We can't spend our time making up for [other] institutions' shortcomings! I mean if I were concerned, if I am a professional in some public institution, and I am faced with this kind of communication issue, I fight to have an interpreter! . . . You may add that we would [be able to] do the same and nothing more! . . . and[,] of course, you close with the classical line, "We remain at your disposal to clarify potential misunderstandings related to cultural representations of illness." . . . We can negotiate that way, without closing the door. Because I am not letting the person out of sight. I want that person to receive the best care he can, starting with the place where he's seen.

When faced with a logic of referrals such as this, Dr. Bennegadi is bound to take a more nuanced rather than normative position, as he had articulated earlier. Here, he clearly backpedaled on his injunction to care for all indiscriminately. His response indicated a sense of indignation, which highlighted a discrepancy between his own moral judgment of the situation—inspired by his personal ideal of clinical responsibility—and the way his colleagues at other institutions handled this situation. At the same time, his ever-present concern about shirking professional responsibility, which I noted in my earlier discussion of transcultural expertise, was also illustrated here when he stated, "I am not letting the person out of sight," or when he feared appearing as though the center were rejecting referring institutions and instructed his colleagues to negotiate peacefully with and not "vex" other institutional actors. This is another classic example of the kinds of double binds experienced by center staff and their anxieties about the triage of patients.

This double bind of expertise, caused when staff at the center wish to refute the logics of a referral while knowing that such refusal might hinder the referred patient's access to health care, was exacerbated by the managerial logics of the health-care system, within which budget restrictions have been consistent since the 1980s (as I explore further in chapter 6). In a hierarchy of health-care needs, the budget for professional interpreters is not a priority and has even been discouraged by some politicians. For example, in 2015, the president of a departmental (county) council in the South of France communicated through national newspaper *Le Figaro* that it would no longer call for interpreters "for patients of foreign origin who consult at medico-social centers." According to him, this type of funding would contribute to the development of "*communautarisme*" (referring to multiculturalism or identity politics): "It is quite unconceivable that our taxes should cover this expenditure. . . . Through our decision, we aim at encouraging the integration of foreigners. This relies on them learning French. . . . Calling for interpreters, on the other hand, would keep these persons excluded" (*Le Figaro* 2015; my translation). From previous research on the role of interpreters in breaking bad news at hospitals (Kotobi, Larchanché, and Kessar 2013), I know that some health professionals adhere to this logic, even when it severely challenges patient-provider communication and thus health-care ethics.

*   *   *

Social representations can travel from one historical and political context to another. In this chapter, the political characterization of migrants is foregrounded as it emerges through state agents' referral narratives. By paying attention to how state agents articulate cultural difference, I have analyzed the ideological aspects of linguistic differentiation (Irvine and Gal 2010). I have looked not only at how ideology contributes to language change, particularly through the evolution of "specialized" mental health care, but also at how it affects boundary production.

In the context of referrals to Centre Minkowska, I have demonstrated that state agents' language, opinions, and actions index migrants as difficult people living in pathological environments, and that they discuss them in language that characterizes their practices as culturally maladaptive while comparing them to local standards. They also use homogenizing language to obscure the variability of migrants' experiences. The language of the referrals I have presented in this chapter reveal logics that relate to state agents' transferal of the responsibility of caring for migrants to other people and agencies. I believe different forms of anxieties underlie this. State agents express individual anxieties that relate to their own experience of not knowing, as well as their often related inability to empathize with patients in the face of complex situations. This, in turn, connects with broader social anxieties around cultural difference in the context of France's ideology, which is based on the idea of cultural unity premised on the use of the French language. In the case of language-based referrals, as with cultural difference-based referrals, the identification of Centre Minkowska as an institution with cultural expertise, offering multilingual mental health support, indirectly cautioned state agents' foregrounding of cultural and linguistic rationales. Identifying whether ideas of cultural or language difference are merely instrumental and related to broader structural constraints proved hard to assess; I return to this in chapter 4.

Regardless of the motives of referring agents, the practical outcome of their decisions was that Minkowska professionals were placed in a double bind, whereby they had to triage an overwhelming number of referrals from other institutions and decide which cases to accept and which they must reject. This complex process generated anxiety for staff at the center and for clinicians in particular; their personal and professional ethics, particularly their drive to help everyone who needs their assistance and their mission of beneficence, fundamentally clashed with practical constraints. What emerged was a willingness to sensitize referring professionals to reconsider their evaluation of situations, either through direct responses to referrals or through accompanying them to work on empathy in transcultural situations.

4 · MANAGING "MIGRANT YOUTH"

Modes of representations of migrant children by French institutional actors act as the "mirror function" (Sayad 1999) to reveal how France approaches the "integration" of its migrant populations. The identification of behavioral problems or learning disabilities in these children—and these two often problematically overlap—is frequently accompanied by discussions on migrant families' socialization model (in reference to French standards) and on what constitutes abnormal behavior/disability. It sheds light on the very categorization of these children as "children of immigrants" or "immigrant youth" as politically and even semantically meaningful—they are commonly referred to as *jeunes issus de l'immigration*, (Simon 2000). Gérard Noiriel points out that the children of Italian, Polish, or Armenian immigrants in France were never categorized in that way (2001, 224); given this, we must question the category as stigmatizing in itself and as contributing to racially homogenize "visible" others (namely "blacks" and "Arabs"). Noiriel (2001) hypothesizes that state "social support" policies (*l'aide sociale*) popularized the category as a way to at once define, diagnose, and solve social ills. This may explain why it is rarely acknowledged as racist—especially in schools (van Zanten 2009), where mechanisms of discrimination are now receiving increasing sociological attention (among them, Brinbaum and Primon 2013; Dubet and Martucelli, 1996; Dubet et al. 2013; Dhume et al. 2011; Felouzis, Favre-Perroton, and Liot, 2005; Felouzis and Fouquet-Chauprade 2015; Ichou and van Zanten 2014; Kleinman 2016; Lorcerie 2011; Payet 1995; van Zanten 2012). It is also first and foremost the result of an assimilationist policy, which promotes exclusionary identity choices.

In the contemporary transcultural clinic, two "problematic" figures emerge in migrant youth referrals. The first relates to second-generation children, whose "double culture" is identified as a risk factor. In that context, expressions of belonging that combine references to both France and a minority culture or a foreign country are perceived negatively, as a conflict of loyalty, potentially leading to social ills and psychological distress among immigrant youth. Until recently, many qualitative studies—in transcultural psychiatry and psychology literature in particular—have provided evidence to counter this, underlying the fact that feelings of exclusion derive instead from France's unwillingness to acknowledge its diversity and to construe it as enriching rather than threatening (Moro 2010). Few sociological studies and surveys reported experiences of discrimination and exclusion among the descendants of migrants (but see Bertossi and Wihtol de Wenden 2007).[1] The second "problematic migrant youth" figure relates to children who recently arrived in France with their families, or arrived unaccompanied, and whose integration into the French education system raises numerous obstacles, mostly related to the acquisition of the French language. The focus on language and learning French as a sign of proper integration is particularly marked in France. The constitution of France as a nation, indivisible, was based on the homogenization of the French language, to the detriment of regional dialects; thus, national ideology is closely intertwined with language proficiency. One could argue that this is the case for all nation-states, but the degree of adhesion to this ideology in France is particularly strong. Mastery of French is thus "iconic" (Irvine and Gal 2000) in that from a linguistic perspective, it inherently signals one's belonging to the nation (Rockwell 2012).

Encounters around school referrals to "specialized" mental health care bring these issues to the fore, as specialists act as experts to mediate between migrant families and cultural representations of French norms. As highlighted in chapter 3, representations of cultural and linguistic difference, equated by referring actors with producing psychopathology, mask structurally related hardships—those encountered by families and their children and those faced by state agents. In this chapter, the testimonies of several professionals, particularly a school psychologist, allow us to better situate these structural constraints and how they shape the logics of referrals to "specialized" mental health institutions like Centre Minkowska. In turn, we will see how, in that context, professionals at Centre Minkowska often resist the demand of institutions, as it culturalizes or pathologizes structural issues.

STARTING SCHOOL: LOCATING "DIFFICULTIES," NAMING DISORDERS AND DISABILITIES

In recent years, schools have become sites for the policing of urban violence—too often associated with children of immigrants. The Base-élève project (Student Basic Information Project), for example, established in 2007, required that information on all children enrolled in kindergarten and primary schools be recorded in a central database, accessible only to heads of schools and city mayors. The official intention was that this would facilitate the general management of schools. The project was highly contested for several reasons, however, including that it initially requested detailed information on children's family members, including nationality, year of arrival in France, native language, and culture of origin. In the summer of 2008, Xavier Darcos, then minister of education, was pressured to remove such data. Today, the files contain limited information, such as a family contact for emergencies and a phone number.

The project was designed in the aftermath of the urban riots of 2005 and 2007, which triggered a national discussion, not so much on the socioeconomic inequalities that were the root cause of such violence but on the management of early delinquency patterns among urban youth. The discussion about delinquency had in fact been initiated well before the riots and had most likely fueled discontent among disadvantaged suburban youth. It had been spurred by the ministry of the interior, then led by Nicolas Sarkozy, leading to the adoption of a law in 2003 on "interior security."[2] That same year, the government had created a parliamentary study group known as the Prevention Commission on Interior Security (Commission prévention sur la sécurité intérieure). The group was headed by moderate right politician Jacques Alain Bénisti and was highly criticized by French intellectuals and school representatives for its preliminary report (Bénisti 2004), which established an implicit relationship between bilingualism among children of immigrants and the risk for delinquency. As a result, it recommended that "foreign parents . . . will have to force themselves to speak French at home so that it becomes the only language for children to express themselves with" (Bénisti 2004, 9, quoted in Muni Toke 2009, 35; my translation). This claim was corrected in 2005, when the group released another version of its report, with a statement that "bilingualism is a great opportunity for a child, unless he or she displays learning disabilities, in which case it becomes an additional complication" (Bénisti 2005, 40; my translation).

Two years later, in 2007, a law related to delinquency was adopted as Loi n° 2007-297 du 5 mars 2007 relative à la prévention de la délinquance.[3] It made schools privileged partners in the institutional detection and prevention of delinquency. Based on equations between education and police surveillance, some school directors chose to oppose their school's participation in the Base-élève project. Other "privileged partners" in the detection and prevention of delinquency were mental health professionals, especially psychiatrists. In the Bénisti report, a section was devoted to psychiatrists' collaboration with schools:

> At the level of kindergarten, it would be useful to design a culture of dialogue with pediatric psychiatrists and teachers, so as to detect very early on any behavior or attitude which could develop into violent behavior or lead the child to fail at school.
>
> Pediatric psychiatrists must be sensitized to the school environment and, alternatively, kindergarten assistants must be sensitized to pediatric psychiatry, so that together they may detect and diagnose children's troubles (*maux*) before making a referral and establishing a broader plan of action (*dispositif*) for prevention around the child. The network of inter-district psychiatry functions well and could be centralized at the departmental level with the establishment of a coordinator.

Children with *difficulties* deserve more attention than others, as early as kindergarten. Therefore it is important to facilitate pediatric psychiatrists' access to schools, in order to facilitate outreach work (*faire un travail de proximité*).

The family physician must also play an important role in the group of referral actors intervening around the child, because he or she is knowledgeable about the family and has their trust (2004, 16; my translation).

This inspired Sarkozy to include a mental health component to his law on delinquency, but under the pressure of the psychiatry community, he was forced to remove it.

This political and legal background underlines, in the detection of behavioral disorders or disabilities among children of immigrants, the interaction between political ideology and the policing of individual behavior through health and educational policies. This problematic interaction emphasizes the shifting line between caring and regulating in specialized mental health care school referrals. I devote the first section of this chapter to school dynamics in the detection of behavioral disorders and disabilities among children of immigrants. I pay particular attention to ways that the recently updated law on disability—theoretically intended to improve care and the school environment for disabled children—triggers conflict situations between school officials and migrant parents. In the second section, I turn to how "specialized" mental health professionals at Centre Minkowska manage school referrals based on behavioral disorder or disability. As I have done in previous chapters, I examine how the center is caught in a double bind, in which its institutional positioning and the very nature of its expertise places it in a position to both amend and contest the dynamics of referrals.

Immigrant descent as the basis of "difficulties"

"Difficulty," as a term of reference in the language of the French education system, is fraught with ambivalence. The term is very vague and could theoretically encompass any problem in any domain. Generally, however, school actors use the word to refer to the fact that a given child is failing at school (*en échec scolaire*); in fact, "student in difficulty" formally replaced "student failing" in the 1980s as part of an effort by the national education system to counteract previous segregating practices, which led to early and arbitrary orientations to special education schools (Monfroy 2002, 33–34). Yet "difficulty" remains ambiguous, as it can potentially refer to different levels of severity in defining academic failure. Consequently, "difficulty" is used as a generic term, capturing concerns as they are initially raised with regard to a given child's problematic school progress before specific causes are identified through psychological and medical assessments. It remains undefined, both in official national education texts and in the professional literature. As a result, naming and identifying become a social process (Monfroy 2002, 34).

When discussing naming and referral practices in chapter 3, I mentioned how "difficulty" as a concept was also often used as a euphemistic and culturally meaningful term that conflated stigmatizing representations of migrants' cultural differences with acknowledgment of the structural inequalities to which they are particularly vulnerable and that may inform their suffering. In this chapter on school referrals, I examine the parallel use of the concept in reference to children of immigrants being "difficult" in the context of the classroom—that is, being either disruptive or absentminded—and presenting a higher incidence of learning "difficulties" for which various diagnoses are later provided. As noted in chapter 3, discussions on the identification of the nature of such "difficulties" often convey stigmatizing representations of immigrants' family structures, lifestyles, and child-rearing practices. More often than not, these are perceived as negatively affecting children's learning abilities and behavior, as identified by schools. Therefore, the connotations of the use of the word in reference to migrants and their children, as well as the racial prejudices and moral comments it implies, require careful attention in the making and naming of school diagnoses, including both learning disabilities and behavioral disorders.

In one case, a referral letter to Centre Minkowska, drafted by a school psychologist of a special education high school, came with exhaustive technical evaluations of the patient-student, provided in separate reports by each of the student's instructors. Although these evaluations clearly establish that the student presents with various learning disabilities, the psychologist emphasizes that "we wish to understand this student's *difficulties* so we can help her as well as we can" (emphasis mine). In the attached letter from the school's director to the district's superintendent, however, formally asking for the student's referral to a special-aid high school, those *difficulties* are clearly summarized. It is specified that after two years spent in middle school, she still could not read or write and, "evidently, could not learn her lessons." Consequently, the student had been transferred to a technical college, where she was being taught leathercraft to make items such as belts and wallets. Again, she was unable to complete the program, for "in addition to the problems already mentioned, she [the student] has *difficulties* with drawing and understanding. She has trouble following guidelines, if she follows them at all. She also displays mild *difficulties* in the manual domain." One might ponder what kind of supplemental information the school might expect from a specialized mental health center, being that the student's learning and motor skill disabilities have been so clearly established, and when the orientation to a special-aid school has already been decided (the district superintendent letter of notification for this decision was included in the patient file).

What alternative *difficulties* does the school psychologist's referral letter allude to that might require cultural expertise of some kind? Nowhere do references to the student's cultural background appear in the patient's file. She was born in France, and the only clue to the student's "cultural difference" was her last name, which suggests that her family is from West Africa, most likely from Ivory Coast or Guinea.[4] What kind of reasoning motivated the school psychologist to link this student's learning disability with her cultural background? I first thought that the psychologist equated the student's parents' cultural difference with a limited ability to offer educational support to their daughter, and difficulties related to navigating the French educational system and following up on their daughter's progress. But then, why would this not be clearly articulated by the psychologist? One would think that so many efforts placed into providing a detailed account of the school situation would be accompanied by an equally detailed rationale on the request for cultural expertise. I had to wonder: Is this what the choice of the word "difficulties" encapsulated? Does the use of such an ambiguous term signal self-censorship in naming the student's cultural difference, or is the relationship between cultural difference and learning disability presumed as common sense, so it does not even have to be articulated? A key question that emerged from my research was whether the word "difficulty," so often mentioned in school referral narratives, acted as a proxy that implied a relationship between school problems and cultural difference.

In his discursive analysis of the construction of a learning-disabled student, Mehan focuses on the "competition over the meaning of ambiguous events . . . play[ing] out in schools every day" as a variety of social actors "try to decide whether a certain child is 'normal' or 'deviant,' belongs in a 'regular educational program' or in a 'special education program'" (1996, 254). In France, the classification of disabilities has become increasingly formalized through state legislation and related institutional reorganization.[5] The goal has been to give the family more agency over the future of their child and over school decision-making, while allowing disabled youth to remain in the least restrictive school environment as possible. However, the administrative management of disabilities at school, from diagnosis to placement, has become increasingly complex and burdensome—despite its intention to improve attendance of disabled children and increase checkups in the diagnostic process. The language of this new system, with its plethora of acronyms, is also difficult to process. School actors, whom I encountered during preclinical consultations or whom I interviewed, themselves complained that they had trouble keeping up, especially as the system's rules evolved constantly.

Seeing one's child diagnosed with a learning disability is a stressful experience for any parent. But with the new legislation, parents' responsibility in taking charge of managing the reported disability burdened them further. Because of the difficulties in communicating in French and because of existing tensions with the school as a state institution, immigrant parents may find themselves in extremely anxiety-ridden situations, in which they understand that the future of their child may be at stake but based on an assessment of the child that they may not understand or with which they may disagree. Conflicts between immigrant parents and school officials thus constantly reoccur around a diagnosis of disability and the special education school transfer. Such conflicts—rather than the diagnosis per se—form the basis of school referrals to specialized mental health centers. But before I turn to analyze how specialized mental health centers manage such conflicts, I first examine how the diagnosis of disability and the referral system is organized in schools.

Disability Representations: The Conflicts between Schools and Migrant Families

During my doctoral fieldwork, I participated in a transcultural psychiatry program, led by Marie Rose Moro at Université Paris 13. In the course of that training, I had the opportunity to meet Murielle, a school psychologist working at a primary school in an eastern suburb of Paris. This suburb hosts a large Malian community, and it had been the site of violent suburban riots involving "migrant youth" in both 2005 and 2007. In the last decade, it has received a lot of attention in the context of new politics of urban planning to improve life in the suburbs. Dilapidated high-rise buildings are being torn down and slowly replaced with low-rise apartment complexes. As we drove to her school, Murielle commented that having nicer buildings would most likely not solve the social issues facing the majority of families in her district.

The suburb is part of a Priority Education Network (REP, Réseau d'éducation prioritaire), formally categorized by the national education system as a Priority Education Zone (ZEP, Zone d'éducation prioritaire), which means that it receives additional funding and autonomy in order to address socially related school problems.[6] REP's goal is to ensure "equal access to school success" (égalité des chances) and to develop partnerships between the school, families, and other related institutions, like social services and CMPs (Dubet 2004).

Murielle described for me what her role as school psychologist was, in the context of the RASED—the Special Aid Network for Students with Difficulties.[7] RASED interventions must take place during school time and must be planned in collaboration with teachers during regular school staff meetings. Parents must be informed of such interventions when their child is involved, and they must provide their agreement for the intervention of a school therapist or psychologist. RASED professionals may not always feel competent addressing a child's difficulties, however; in this case, external consultations can take place. This is how— with children of immigrants, for example—the network can be short-circuited and children sent to specialized health institutions, like Centre Minkowska.

Teachers and psychologists employed in the RASED program address problems from kindergarten to elementary schools exclusively. Each RASED team is typically in charge of all schools in one geographically defined school district. A RASED team consists of a special-aid teacher in charge of learning disabilities (maître E), a special-aid teacher in charge of "socialization/relational" disabilities (maître G), and a school psychologist.[8] This wide range of specialized support, from pedagogical to psychological, is also perceived as preventive in nature. As one school psychologist explained to me: "As soon as children—and potentially their families—are identified as having difficulties with school—whether it is *a problem of cultural adaptation,* of understanding what the institution expects from them, or simply of wanting to learn—we can coordinate *an intervention* to prevent problems from worsening. The goal is also to encourage sharing perspectives and partnership between the various professional actors in the school system. Ultimately, this should lead to the best adapted response to any kind of problem" (emphases mine). Once a disability has been diagnosed, the school psychologist must meet with the child's family in order to report the disability and decide on a transfer to a special education institution. CLIS classes, for example, are school inclusion classes (*classes d'inclusion scolaire*), located within primary schools, which provide for a small group of children (twelve maximum) presenting with some kind of disability. Some CLIS classes are structured to respond to a specific impairment—mental, auditory, visual, or motor. CLIS classes thus assist children who are considered unable to integrate into an ordinary class on their own. They provide these children with individualized teaching while allowing them to partake in the school's collective pedagogical projects with the rest of the pupils. Depending on the level of his or her disability, a child can spend some time in "regular" classes, where he or she can follow the general curriculum at his or her own pace.

Until the adoption of a law on the rights of disabled persons in February 2005 (Loi pour l'égalité des droits et des chances, la participation et la citoyenneté des personnes handicappées), referrals to CLIS classes were decided by a special education commission (District Commission for Pre-elementary and Elementary Education), with the agreement of the child's family. Out of concern for the social isolation and social reintegration of "disabled" pupils, new conditions were added to performing such referrals, which gave greater involvement to health structures attending to the child's disability and to the child's family. Since the beginning of the 2006 school year, families must fill out the file for referral to disability structures on their own.

MDPH structures (Departmental Houses for Disabled Persons) were created to discuss the referral propositions and grant or deny approval. Following initial acknowledgment of a disability-related referral, a second round of approvals must be granted by the Commission on the Rights and Autonomy of Disabled Persons on the one hand, and by the health-care structure monitoring the child for his or her disability on the other.[9] An individualized "project" (School Success Personalized Project) is then proposed to the family, which has to grant final approval for the referral. Depending on enrollment availabilities in the child's school district, the school superintendent assigns the child to a specific class.

Teachers in charge of CLIS classes have received specialized training, and they work in close collaboration with the school's "pedagogical team" and, ideally, with health-care structures assisting their pupils.[10] At the secondary level, the equivalents to CLIS classes are Regional Establishments for Adapted Teaching and Adapted Sections for General and Professional Teaching, but these are located outside regular secondary schools and emphasize individual professional or technical training for disabled children. Murielle describes her role as a school psychologist in this complex referral system. Together with maître G, she works on "socialization/relational" disabilities. She explains that until recently, the school was in charge of seeking out MDPH directly to report a disability case. Today, this responsibility falls on parents' shoulders. Murielle shares her uneasiness about this transfer of responsibility. Although the policy is intended to foster families' autonomy, it is apparent, through Murielle's experience, that often a decision has already been made by the school, and that families are under heavy pressure to both accept the disability diagnosis and submit a disability file with the MDPH. "It requires a lot of patience and tenacity," she says. "The most difficult thing is to constantly have to mediate between the child's parents and the administration. Often, the administration pushes for a mental health referral, so they can get rid of a complicated situation." Noting my interest in her comments and work experience, she invited me to attend an appointment with the Malian father of an eight-year-old child, still enrolled in kindergarten (typically enrolling ages three through six) and diagnosed with autism.

Before Mr. Diarra arrived, Murielle explained the situation to me. Salif, Mr. Diarra's son, was diagnosed with autism four years before, at the end of his first year in kindergarten. Autism is a tricky diagnosis, since there are no medical tests for it. A diagnosis must be based on observation of the individual's communication, behavior, and developmental levels. To complicate things further, many of the behaviors associated with autism are shared with other disorders, such as developmental delays, behavioral disorders, or hearing disability. Therefore, detecting autism can take time. Murielle explained to me that Salif would rarely make eye contact with people, had an extremely limited vocabulary and mostly articulated sounds, and would isolate himself, as if drawn into his own world. At the end of Salif's first year in kindergarten, the Diarra family was called to school by the director to discuss an alternative school program for Salif. The school had established a part-time program for children with disabilities (CLIS), which Salif was eligible to attend. Following the law of February 2005, the conditions of schooling for disabled children must be adapted so that educational and therapeutic needs are complementary. How a child's schooling is organized is presumably undertaken through consultations between the family, the school, and health-care professionals; a personalized program is then developed based on a precise evaluation of the child's needs, and it is regularly reviewed and revised. Generally, the child is accommodated with part-time schooling alternating with specialized care.

Unfortunately, at the time Salif's case was discussed, the alternative program had reached its maximum of pupils enrolled. The school's director therefore approached the Diarras with the possibility that their son be sent to a medical-educational institution separate from the school (IME, Institut médico-educatif). Salif's father was opposed to the idea. His son was "special," he told the school director, but certainly not disabled. He had had a spell cast on him (*marabouté*) the day he was born. His mind was governed by a *jinn*, who would not let go of him. Salif's father believed that one day, his son would come back to his own self, free from the spirit in his head, and things would be normal. In fact, Murielle explained to me, the parents had consulted with a multitude of diviners (*marabouts*) in Paris with the hope of finding the right "cure" for their son.

Almost four years had passed since the first meeting between the Diarras and the school director without their being able to reach an agreement on Salif's schooling. During that time, Murielle had acted as a mediator between them. On several occasions, the school director had threatened the Diarras with a lawsuit for child maltreatment. Murielle had successfully gained more time from the director at each threat, convincing her that the Diarras needed time to come to terms with the situation, and that it was in Salif's best interest to let his parents be part of the decision-making process. In addition to meetings with Mr. Diarra to deal with the administrative conundrum that Salif's case had become, Murielle also saw Mrs. Diarra on a regular basis. Murielle suspected that Mrs. Diarra had suffered from severe postpartum depression following Salif's birth. She had shared with Murielle her difficulties relating to her son and confessed that she often simply left him sitting in front of the TV, where he would be so absorbed by the images that she would not have to deal with him.

A few months before my visit to Murielle's school, the situation had shifted. Murielle was to meet with Mr. Diarra to discuss family changes and Salif's progress, and he had decided to finally sign on to the personalized program adapted by the MDPH for Salif. The appointment had been difficult to schedule, since Mr. Diarra worked long, ever-changing shifts as a janitor at Charles de Gaulle airport, and travel time from home to work was lengthy. When he arrived, Murielle asked his permission for me to sit in on their meeting, and he agreed. He was eager to tell Murielle about the trip his whole family had undertaken to Mali, with Salif and their newborn child. It was his and his wife's first time back home since they had come to France. The trip was transformative for the family on many levels, including Salif's behavior. Mr. Diarra had taken Salif to "the bush" (*la brousse*), where they visited a renowned ritual specialist. The latter had prescribed the family a variety of herbal remedies, some to be mixed with food and liquids, others to be mixed with Salif's bathwater. Every night, Salif was administered a ritual bath, and within a week, he seemed to display significant behavioral changes, making efforts at uttering complete sentences and making eye contact more regularly. Mr. Diarra commented:

I think the *jinn* has left, finally. You know, when I think about all the money I invested in those *marabouts* (ritual specialists) here in France . . . I know people say they're all charlatans, but when you're in our situation, you try everything. [Turning to me] You know, if it was not for Murielle, I don't know what would have happened with Salif. I know people at school mean well for him, but as his parents, don't we know best? People have been so mean to us at times. Only Murielle took the time to listen to us, me and my wife also. She understands. [Turning back to Murielle] Thank you, really.

After Mr. Diarra left, Murielle took advantage of school recess to take me to the kindergarten section of the school so I could meet Salif. When I saw him, he was playing ball with one of the school assistants. Although he seemed to lack agility and coordination, he appeared very engaged in the game itself—throwing the ball back and forth—although he did not always seem to intend to throw the ball back to the assistant. Murielle interrupted them to take Salif to a reading room, where she observed him play with a variety of plastic objects. She then had him sit between the two of us, and we flipped through the pages of a children's book, paying attention to how he engaged with the content. At one point, he stopped and pointed at the drawing of a mountain and, aloud, articulated *"Montagne!"* (Mountain!). Murielle turned to me with a look of amazement. "See, he never ceases to amaze me. He appears to have such a limited vocabulary, and yet he regularly comes [up] with these words out of nowhere."

Diagnoses of disability may sometimes be very difficult to establish. This may be related to the very nature of the disability, as with autism in Salif's case. In school, it is not the existence of the disability that is so problematic—be it related to mental, auditory, visual, or motor skills. Rather, it is the severity of the disability and how to deal with it that becomes more complicated. As Salif's case illustrates, the difficulty also resides in communicating the disability to immigrant parents and negotiating the potentially divergent explanations parents may have about the disability and its origins. Schools may not always be willing to take the time to accept such negotiations. Were it not for Murielle's personal engagement with the Diarras and her sensibility to their conflict with the school, Salif's parents may have been brought to court and Salif most likely placed in foster care by child services. A referral to a specialized mental health center would certainly have taken place.

What Salif's case highlights is the rigidity that institutional actors often readily display with migrants or their children, which ineluctably creates conflicting situations where there should not be any—or at least where they could be easily avoided. The Diarra family was fortunate to find someone like Murielle to mediate for them. Her willingness to listen and be receptive to the family was essential in unlocking this situation and avoiding Salif's referral to a specialized mental health center, where the same dispositions—listening, tolerance, and hospitality—would have been offered. Communicating acted as a substitute for referral and a potential lawsuit.

BEHAVIORAL DISORDERS: THE CONFLICTS
BETWEEN TEACHERS AND CHILDREN OF IMMIGRANTS

I have described the intricacies of negotiating the representations of a child's diagnosed disability between school officials and migrant families. A second challenge related to the detection of "difficulties" among children of immigrants in schools is linked to the impact of broader racial and ethnic prejudices on child-teacher interactions. In that respect, one category, which seems to plague children of immigrants, appears particularly problematic: the behavioral disorder category.

When I asked Murielle to tell me which obstacles children of migrants commonly face at school, and which may lead them to be referred to a special-aid school, she identified language (which teachers often explained as the result of family members not speaking French at home) and behavioral disorders. To Murielle, those labeled "behavioral disorders" were most problematic with respect to children of migrants. She addressed how such diagnoses may be culturally biased and discriminatory, imposing an etiology of pathology that is imbued by racial and ethnic prejudices on generic African lifestyles and family arrangements: "If you will, behavioral disorders, teachers interpret it that way: 'It's normal, it's a migrant's child, from a polygamous family, the mother doesn't master the French language.' So it's all the clichés they put into it." She also commented on teachers' rigidity when it comes to adapting to situations related to different cultural practices. She recalled an incident during which a young boy, who had shaved his head for a Muslim religious ceremony, was sent out of the classroom because he refused to take his hat off:

> That was nothing. . . . It could have been defused in ten seconds by the teacher, and in fact, it was a detail for her which took huge proportions . . . because it was . . . for her it was the lack of respect for the teacher, when it was not that at all. It was an 11-year-old child who didn't want to show his shaved head . . . so the proportions it took is that the teacher would not accept him in the classroom, the child was not allowed to cross the entrance door, so he fled to the playground, he jumped over the fence. . . . He didn't understand either . . . and so I talked with him for 30 minutes, and when I took him back to the classroom, the teacher said, "I don't want him anymore." So it's violent. I received it very violently. And I thought to myself, "How does *he* interpret that?"

When I asked Murielle why, in her opinion, teachers respond differently to children of migrants in the classroom, she mentioned cultural discrepancies between children and teachers, but she also emphasized the negative impact of teachers' representations of these children as being threatening suburban thugs: "I think that the migrant child scares teachers, so automatically they show greater resistance, whereas a child . . . a French child . . . there's not this feeling of discrepancy. The teacher feels more at ease. The teacher is scared I think. Especially in the CM2 (fifth grade) with the older ones. The teacher is afraid, and so automatically he is more rigid." In reference to the boy who had shaved his head, she continued, "The teacher has a lot of *fantasies*. So the teacher told me, 'This child will be dangerous.' So I ask her, 'So just like that, we're going to report him to social services because, potentially, in two years, he will be *difficult*?' See, it's ridiculous. Many things are being projected" (emphases mine). Stigmatizing projections thus shape teachers' categorization of children of migrants as "difficult" children (difficulty broadly related to their migrant status), bound to become "children in difficulty" (difficulty acknowledged as related to a disability).

Although it did not focus on cultural or racial stigmatization in relation to children of migrants at school, in her study on the definition of students in difficulty in ZEPs, Monfroy found that "students from lower social classes are frequently perceived [by their teachers] through very generic representations, massively resorting to images of deprivation and social misery, as well as to explanations framed in terms of 'sociocultural disability'" (2002, 35). Teachers' representations focused on students' behavior and attitude rather than on academic performance strictly, with a strong propensity to psychologize problems. These attributions, which are external to the school context, lead teachers to commonly categorize students in difficulty in two broad categories: withdrawal (*figure "du retrait"*) or resistance (*figure "de la résistance"*) (Monfroy 2002, 36). Similar categorizations are used with children of migrants in France, as case studies in this chapter demonstrate. Monfroy also shows how such external attributions lead teachers to "consider children's difficulties as being unrelated to pedagogy and/or school, but rather from a lack of will, of interest, or of motivation, sometimes a pathological problem (paralysis—*"un blocage"*), on which they cannot act because they would be related to these students' personal characteristics and/or their families" (Monfroy 2002, 37). Again, one may easily understand how stigmatizing stereotypes about migrants' unusual family structures and lifestyles—and the dangerous youth they purportedly breed—would make children of migrants particularly vulnerable to such categorizations.

Murielle commented that there were contradictions between teachers' negative responses to children of migrants and the fact that they chose to work in a ZEP district, in which they would most likely have to deal with such demographics in the classroom. She hypothesized that for some, it was the motivation to stay related to a colonial-like feeling of "standing above" (*on se sent au-dessus*) or feeling all-powerful: "If those same teachers went to a school in a bourgeois neighborhood, they wouldn't have the same reactions. Because the kinds of reactions they have in a ZEP, parents wouldn't accept that." According to Murielle, among the youngest teachers, turnover is quite common. Those who stay may find their work conditions arduous, which negatively affects both their mental health and their relationship with students: "I'm telling you about teachers who have been there for over 10 years. Who feel bad, who are depressed on top of that. So the child faces depressed persons who react violently at some times, but who stay nonetheless in the ZEP. Whereas we . . . well, I chose. I chose the ZEP."

In her study on the definition of students in difficulty in ZEPs, Monfroy concluded that teachers' distress and professional burnout weigh significantly in their subjective assessment of such students, and the consequences that derive from such assessment (withdrawing their responsibility from the situation, referring the case to the RASED team, requesting a transfer to a special education school) (2002, 39). All these reasons make referrals for children of migrants particularly problematic.

Murielle came back to the ambivalence of making families responsible for managing the referral themselves in such contexts. While she acknowledged that the goal of the reform was to enable families to become the decision-makers in relation to their child's disability, it completely overlooked families' needs and constraints in doing so, including language barriers, cultural representations of the disability, and other obstacles related to administrative intricacies (filling out the disability form and deciphering the jargon and acronyms of the special education network): "*Even [for] a French family*, it's very, very hard, see, to refer a child, to elaborate a super complicated case. Me, they come to work on the file with me, I don't understand anything. Frankly, the formulas, the boxes to check . . . And on top of that, there are their representations. For them, their child is not sick . . . not deficient. It's something else. . . . It's nice to give them responsibilities, but they need to be accompanied, and I'm afraid to get involved in . . . to betray . . . to betray."

Murielle's feeling of betrayal was linked to the institutional conundrum she faced, of being trusted with a mission to deal with complex situations while being deprived of the means to accomplish this mission. In this context, children of migrants were more vulnerable than others, both because their families lacked the resources to manage their disability and because the professionals themselves lacked the proper tools to evaluate the disability: "And so . . . what's characteristic is those children of migrants who are referred . . . uh . . . I mean you go to a CLIS, if you will, in my district, out of 12 children, you have 10 blacks (*tu as dix "blacks"*). And our tests, uh, well, even though it's the WISC-IV, I find it to be more and more cognitive. I find it to evaluate children poorly. So evidently, we have children who are labeled as deficient, and . . . that hurts me too."[11]

Murielle's personal and professional ethics were being affected by a procedure that generates unequal treatment and stigma. However, this motivated her to resist stigmatizing and unmotivated disability referrals. Together with other RASED colleagues, Murielle developed strategies to reduce the number of referrals of students with a possible disability to MDPH from an average of twelve under her predecessor to two referrals a year. Such strategies included not following procedures by the letter, taking time to examine situations among referring partners, and communicating with the family:

> It is said in the texts that when you have a doubt, *a doubt*, you can make a referral [emphasis hers]. Uh . . . I think a doubt is not sufficient because it can cause a lot of damage. So I wouldn't say I expect facts either, because sometimes, uh . . . but it has to be prepared, and it's prepared with the family. . . . Now all the education teams come to see me, and we discuss the referral again, what's positive, what's negative, what it can entail, and then I inform the parents. Always, always . . . that was my objective, that was my big work three years ago, and now, with social services, I have positive feedback. They tell me "Ah, it's nice because now, referrals, there are less of them, it's carefully examined," so for them it's easier after that to work with the family.

Murielle's professional testimony highlights the importance of establishing a respectful dialogue between school actors and migrant families as a way to avoid arbitrary referrals as well as biased diagnoses, which may negatively and unfairly affect the future school trajectories for the children of migrants. This is especially true of behavioral disorder diagnoses, for which the assessment is relatively subjective. Murielle dedicates much of her time and energy to acting as a safeguard in the establishment of such assessments. Disability diagnoses, on the other hand, subject to a series of broader institutional assessments—both medical and educational—are less likely to form the basis of an arbitrary referral, even though some disabilities are more difficult to measure objectively than others. For these cases, the negotiation of the diagnosis itself with the family is most problematic, and this may hinder an appropriate therapeutic response. Migrant parents may indeed provide culturally different explanations for their child's disability, as Salif's case illustrates.

FROM SCHOOLS TO CENTRE MINKOWSKA: CIRCULATING AND CONTESTING

In this second part of this chapter, I examine how the staff of specialized mental health services become involved in the negotiation of diagnoses of disorder or disability for the children of migrants. On what basis is their professional expertise involved? What is their position vis-à-vis schools' decisions? How do they apprehend the relation between cultural difference and the presence or development of a disorder or disability among the children of migrants? To what extent do they or can they contest the stigmatizing nature of referrals and related interpretations of migrant youth suffering?

Individual School Actor Referral

Marie-Jo called me to attend a pre-consultation meeting with a school assistant, Sabine, who had called Centre Minkowska about the possibility of referring a child from one of the district's schools.[12] When Marie-Jo asked Sabine how she had heard about the center, she responded that she had done her own research and had found the center online. The center's description led her to think that it would respond appropriately to the needs of a pupil her school has been concerned about. Therefore, she had taken it on herself to call the center and set up an appointment.

Sabine first asked Marie-Jo to introduce the center and detail its activities. Marie-Jo launched into a lengthy presentation, beginning with the history of the center, from its creation in the 1950s to respond to the health needs of postwar asylum seekers, to its evolution into a center guided by a clinical medical anthropology approach. "This orientation," she explained, "takes into account culture in therapy, without falling to the extreme of defining all pathologies as culturally determined. It also seeks to avoid denying the influence of culture altogether, which eventually leads to racism and ethnocentrism. What the center does is that it takes into account the cultural nature of the clinical encounter between two explanatory models—that of the patient, and that of the clinician." She made references, in English, to the concepts of "disease," "illness," and "sickness" as used by the center in its institutional presentation. "This perspective on mental health allows clinicians to maintain their own theoretical orientation, whether Freudian, Lacanian, constructivist, et cetera."

Following Marie-Jo's presentation, Sabine proceeded to present the case of a third-grade pupil, Anais, the daughter of Mauritian migrants. Sabine explained that she had recently attended a school staff meeting with the school psychologist, Anais's teacher, and "the rest of the staff in charge of pupils in difficulty at school." She had heard the teacher report that Anais had trouble keeping up in class, and that it was difficult for her to understand assignments and even stories. Her grades were falling, and her vocabulary was very limited. She was very shy in the classroom, but sometimes she behaved violently with her schoolmates during recess. Sabine said she had observed pupils making fun of her: "She's really stupid," one of them said in front of the teacher during recess. Anais had already had "problems" in kindergarten, and the school had her repeat her third and last grade (*grande section*). "When she went to primary school, no one followed her development, and now, no one wants her to repeat a class again," Sabine added. After the staff meeting, she went to talk to Anais's teacher and told her that perhaps she could pay more attention to the little girl and try to make her look good in front of the other pupils. She informed us that Anais was often absent from school. During the first school trimester alone, she had been absent nineteen times, her mother alternately reporting Anais's stomach pains, headaches, or fever. "To me," Sabine said, "all of those are psychosomatic symptoms, you know."

Sabine had then decided to schedule a meeting with Anais's mother directly. No one else at school had bothered to do so, she pointed out. She had heard Anais's teacher mention that perhaps Anais's mother was an alcoholic (although, according to Sabine, the teacher had never met the mother). "As far as I'm concerned," she continued, "I suspect there might be conjugal violence behind all of this." Marie-Jo nodded. Sabine went on to explain that Anais's mother was a stay-at-home mom, who had arrived in France in 1991. Her father was a house painter, but she had never met him. They also had a son, born in 2001, who was failing at school as well, "which strengthens my suspicion that there may be a problem at home. The day I visited her mother at their home," she continued, "Anais seemed very happy that someone had come out of concern about her. But the mother appeared very reticent when I spoke to her about psychotherapy for Anais. You're gonna have to take it slow with them!" she warned Marie-Jo.

This meeting took place in early April. When Marie-Jo called the center's secretary to schedule an appointment, there was nothing available before the end of the month. Sabine seemed very disappointed. However, Marie-Jo readily reassured her, telling her that she had made a good decision referring Anais to the center, and that they would use this first appointment to assess the situation. "I agree," Marie-Jo said, "that Mauritian families often display very rigid family structures, accompanied with conjugal violence. Perhaps we can investigate this option as a key to explain this child's school problems. Also, in these families, people often try and make sense of their children's school failure. They look for outside explanations—sorcery, for example—which could influence the child's behavior and therefore explain problems at school." Marie-Jo then asked Sabine whether she would be willing, as the referring person, to accompany Anais and her mother at the center on the day of the appointment. "Well . . . I don't have much time off. . . . I already took . . . my free time to come here and try to help this family. I have a family of my own, you know," Sabine replied, looking at her agenda. "No, I don't think I'll be able to make it for that appointment."

After the appointment was scheduled and Sabine had left the room, I stayed with Marie-Jo to gain her impressions of the meeting. I asked her about the weight of the school's cultural representation of Anais's parents on the child's academic difficulties. She quickly responded that there might indeed be a true learning disability, without any issue with the family. But what she seemed most concerned about was Sabine's behavior and her unwillingness to go out of her way to accompany Anais and her family at the center. "She bothers reporting the situation to us, and then she won't come here to help solve it!" she said, irritated. "It's the same with social workers. We apply rules under the pretense of exploring situations with people and help them solve their problems. For example, a lot of social workers confronted with quarrels among polygamous families refer women to shelters, without even bothering to speak to their husband first. I mean, everyone knows the husband is a central figure in the African family! Then they act surprised when women come back to their husbands after a week, without the root problem being solved! This is why so many migrants hate social workers!"

The appointment was rescheduled earlier than planned due to a cancellation, and two weeks later Anais came to the center with her mother and younger brother. Marie-Jo invited me to attend the consultation. Before we entered the room, she told me that Sabine had called her to let her know that the situation seemed to have greatly improved at school after the teacher had decided to focus her attention on Anais. With the help of the school psychologist, the teacher had made efforts to boost Anais's self-confidence, both in private meetings and in the classroom. Since then, everything seemed to have gotten "back into order." And indeed, the consultation with the family was very short. Anais's mother said that she had no problem to report concerning school. Anais concurred, smiling, and when asked by Marie-Jo, she responded briefly that she liked school and her teacher. Marie-Jo tried at various instances to elicit information concerning Anais's mother's immigration story, her husband's work, and her life at home. The mother gave her straightforward, factual answers, giving me the impression that while appreciating Marie-Jo's concern, she was unsure how these questions related to her little girl. Meanwhile, her six-year-old son jumped up and down restlessly, constantly pulling his mother's hand to stroke his face. After the family left and we exited the room, Marie-Jo turned to me and declared, "Surely there was no need for a psychological follow-up here. . . . The little boy, on the other hand . . . I wonder if he could use some therapy!"

This case is particularly interesting, as the referral came from an individual initiative: Sabine took the initiative to help Anais and her family. It is unclear whether her individual referral effort resulted from the cultural reading she had made of the situation or whether she seriously suspected violence at home and framed her referral vaguely in cultural terms to access an outside intervention. Lack of institutional resources may have motivated Sabine, more so than cultural bias. But what this case more clearly shows is Marie-Jo's imposition of a cultural interpretation of the situation when she suggested that "Mauritian families often display very rigid family structures, accompanied with conjugal violence." In that respect, she acted in complete contradiction to the center's ethos. Meanwhile, Marie-Jo contested Sabine's intervention on the basis that she had decided to manage a "problem" without personally engaging with it. Marie-Jo's parallel to social workers' detrimental interventions among African families translates her critique of institutional actors' intrusive and inappropriate behavior, lacking sensitivity to what she thinks are well-known cultural rules. As a transcultural professional, Marie-Jo appears to have wanted to explore the possibility of a clinical consultation for Anais, and therefore she assumed the existence of relevant cultural dynamics underlying Anais's potential learning disability. By doing so, she placed herself in a double-bind situation in which, despite the lack of relevant cultural factors in

Anais's case, her institutional expertise led her to adopt a cultural relativist stance and feel obliged to pursue the case with a clinical intervention.

The Double Culture Issue

Marie, a TEF at Minkowska, opened the MEDIACOR meeting. On that day, the referral tackled the thorny issue of "double culture," the very formulation of which reveals France's ambivalence toward multiculturalism and mixed identities. From a clinical perspective, the process of identity elaboration for children whose parents are first-generation migrants may trigger intrapsychic conflict—particularly during adolescence (Idriss 2009; Moro 2010). But the notion of double culture as used by social actors often problematizes mixed identity as a threat to Frenchness and as a potentially pathological process. Marie commenced by introducing the case of Ibrahim, a fifteen-year-old French boy, who evidently speaks French and is said to be "of Senegalese origin." He lives at home with his parents and his three younger brothers. His parents are Guinean, but their families live in Senegal. He was referred to Centre Minkowska by an educator at the Juvenile Judicial Protection Service in Paris on the grounds of what the educator described as a "double culture" issue. The educator had been seeing Ibrahim for a year in relation to an alleged crime, about which he knows only that no judgment has been made.

In the following, I present a series of exchanges among the psychiatrists, the social worker, the attending TEFs, and me about the legal context in order to locate the referral and Centre Minkowska's role. Marie continues quoting the educator, who claims that "the transmission of values from Ibrahim's parents and the issue of the double culture are at stake in Ibrahim's power attitude. For that reason, it seems necessary to us that he, together with his family, can clarify Ibrahim's position in their family and his plural identity." From the remainder of the referral letter, we gather that Ibrahim does not acknowledge any kind of authority, be it judicial, parental, or educational. The only thing he wants to do is go back to Senegal, where he met his extended family a year ago. And the parents, and Ibrahim himself, are very interested in the issue of complex identities, and they would like to know more about it, including, as his educator put it, "this African part of him."

At that point, Dr. Bennegadi invites participants to ask questions about the case. We conclude that we lack the necessary information to justify the fact that Ibrahim's case was referred to the Juvenile Judicial Protection Service. Still, we are intrigued about the focus on Ibrahim's "double culture," and we debate it:

DR. B: Please give your arguments and listen to one another. This is a highly complex debate. It is important to know what we are talking about. Let's validate, or counter argue this notion of . . . She pronounced sentences that are very important to deconstruct. . . . He supposedly has a double culture. . . . This is not like referring to a harmonious biculturalism. Rather, she interprets that as a schizophrenic conflict. And this African part of him, we have to find it!

DR. C: Is this African part brought up because there is a conflict with authority, and authority is here in France, with his parents? Is it brought up here and now precisely because there is a problem with authority, and more so with the law, or was it something which was indeed ... well as soon as he rediscovered his roots, following that trip? ...

DR. B: OK, let's talk psychology. You are referring to the superego, and to the organization of the ego at 15. In general, what happens at 15, whatever the culture?

TEF: The confrontation with the identity, the father's identity, and with the law.

DR. B: All right, from this structuration of the ego, what we call "affiliations" are implemented. He is 15. All that we heard from the educator ... it's hard to hear anything else but "he is Senegalese, he is Senegalese, he is Senegalese. Culture, Africa. Culture, Africa." As if ... at the end, we are starting to understand that he transgresses because he is African.

. . .

ME: Regardless, it is possible to say that, at the time of adolescence, and in an intercultural context, the transition from filiation to affiliation can raise loyalty conflicts, issues that may be considered as specific to this intercultural context, even though there is no indication of that in the letter ...

DR. B: I would reformulate what you just said: it is not specific to the intercultural context but specific to this boy, who expresses it with references belonging to multiple registers ...

ME: Well, actually, we don't know what he expresses ...

DR. B: Well, that is, he has the right to position himself as the eldest of an African family, just as he has the right to claim he is French! This is not where the pathology is located. The pathology is related to who he is in the eye of the other. With his crime, he positioned himself in a situation of stigmatization. And our colleague adheres to that script out of goodwill ... out of goodwill, thinking that she identified an internal conflict related to the confrontation of two cultures. These are highly foggy formulations. We do not know anything about this boy! ... So we don't know anything, besides that someone tells us there are bad feelings related to cultural difference. Please let us know what's going on. Here is how making references belonging to two different registers or to multiple registers is turned into pathology.

. . .

ME: What about inviting the team to come and meet us?

DR. B: Yes. That is what I wanted to hear. We will invite the team to come and meet us so we can debate things with them, and help them realize that either they have transgressed from an anthropological perspective, or that the boy is tough, that he manipulates, on the one hand pretending to be French, on the other, asserting that he is not, that he resorts to complex manipulative strategies ... in which case we must be able to bring up a psychological perspective, rather than an exoticizing ethnological interpretation. For at present, what do we know? Do we have clues? Have you identified any semiology clues, like sleep disorders, behavioral disorders? Does he have food disorders, does he cut himself, does he use weed? Have you heard any of that? . . . So let's have the team come and talk about Ibrahim, and we'll see what turns out.

In the end, we never met Ibrahim. His educator called us to let us know that Ibrahim had left on vacation and that he did not see the relevance of coming to meet us.

For Minkowska professionals, the situation remained unclear. While we did make efforts to apply a culturally sensitive approach to the referral, it appeared that the weight of cultural representations put to the forefront in the referral letter hid a much more complex situation, one that most likely related to communication challenges between the institution, the family, and the adolescent himself; the latter's response to the referral seemed to confirm that was the case. In their ethnography of a house for adolescents (*maison des adolescents*)—which, like Centre Minkowska, receives referrals from a range of state institutions serving children and adolescents (schools, child protection services, and so on), a great proportion of them from migrant families—French sociologists Isabelle Coutant and Jean-Sébastien Eideliman (2013) show how institutional interventions themselves may destabilize family dynamics, either positively or negatively, so that, depending on the nature of the problems and family dynamics, adolescents may resist or appropriate, at times even instrumentalize, mental health professionals' help.

Integrating Recent Migrants and "Learning Difficulties"

We received a referral from the education team of a Parisian high school, calling our attention to the situation of a few of their students enrolled in a UPE2A class (Pedagogical Unit for Arriving Non-francophone Pupils), a class designed to welcome newly arrived, non-French-speaking students or children in traveling situations (*enfants du voyage*—referring to children whose parents are traveling, or to Roma children specifically) who require intensive teaching in French. "Since the beginning of the school-year," the letter stated, "we noticed that a few students face major difficulties in making progress on various subjects, which appear to us as 'cognitive difficulties.' Their behaviors and the obstacles they meet in the context of learning, in part related to their experience among other things, let us believe that they could benefit from psychological support. Considering they are non-French-speaking students, it is difficult for us to find a center that accepts . . . them[,] and this is why we turn to you."

In recent years, with the refugee crisis and the increasing number of unaccompanied minors, we have received a great deal of these types of referrals. Education professionals—including those trained to work in UPE2A classes—sometimes feel helpless in providing the proper support and attention students need. The most challenging part may be the orientation. Each child acquires French at a different speed. Some have lived traumatic experiences on their way to France and require greater support than their teacher can provide. Language obstacles may make it difficult for the teacher to identify such needs; alternatively, a wide range of (often behavioral) difficulties encountered in the context of the classroom—agitation, lack of concentration, introversion—will be readily interpreted through the lens of psychopathology.

The first training and information centers for the schooling of migrant children (Centres de formation et d'information pour la scolarisation des enfants de migrants) were created in 1975 to train teachers to integrate these children into mainstream schools. Until the 1980s, the policies of these centers were rather ambiguous, as the goal of integration was mixed with a need to preserve contact with the culture of origin in the light of prospective return migration (Schiff 2012, 112). In 1990, the centers' mission was broadened with the creation of ZEPs. What this did was make official a practice that had been going on since the 1980s, which consisted of grouping together newly arrived children and the children of resident migrants who were failing at school due to a lack of social integration. While the creation of ZEPs did not label any groups, it implicitly targeted them (Schiff 2012, 113). In 2002, academic centers for the schooling of newly arrived migrant children and children from the Roma community were created, with the objective of implementing individualized progressive education through specialized pedagogical units (UPE2A) (Ministère de l'éducation nationale et de la jeunesse 2012). Unfortunately, these centers have encountered both resistance and lack of interest from school administrations, thus ultimately placing the success of UPE2A classes on the individual practices and personal engagement of some teachers (Schiff 2012, 113). As Schiff comments, "The individualized integration system clearly raises the issue of a tension between a necessary differential treatment and an integration ideal that in the end 'does not make a difference'" (2012, 120).

Let me return to the referral. This was the first of its kind in that it introduced us to no less than five different students potentially needing psychological support. All of them were boys, four of them aged sixteen and one aged eighteen. For each one of them, the team had written a short descriptive paragraph of the situation:

> Mohamed is 18, from Burkina Faso. He speaks Mooré. He never went to school before, even in his country of origin. He arrived in France a year ago, under extremely trying conditions, and he often display anxiety signs. He lives alone, without his family. He lacks consistency when he speaks, and he is quite introverted. He isolates himself, shows difficulties blending in with the rest of the students, and (shows difficulties in) organizing. Sometimes, he has "mental

block" moments, during which he freezes for long minutes without watching nor speaking to anyone.

Mamadou is 16, from Mali. He speaks Bambara. He was not schooled in his country of origin, and his immigration trajectory was very long and painful. He now lives alone in France, without his family. As far as his schooling, he shows major cognitive problems and his progress is close to nil. He lacks concentration in the classroom and sometimes he has rapid mood swings: he can go from being joyful to displaying great sadness. This boy really seems lost.

Souleymane is 16, from Mali. He speaks Bambara. Like the previous two students, he is alone in France and his migration journey was traumatic. He barely communicates with other students in the class, even with those who speak his mother tongue, and keeps physically isolated from others. He shows poor hygiene and self-neglect—perhaps related to hydrophobia. As far as schooling, he makes very little progress.

Zyed is 16, from Tunisia. His mother tongue is Arabic. He lives with his family. Although he went to school in his country of origin, he shows serious learning difficulties and disturbing speech and language impairments, which considerably slow down his school progress, despite him being assiduous and persevering. His father is favorable to his son getting care from you, and anxiously awaits our help.

Yazid is 16, from the Comoros. He lives with his father and brothers and sisters. He seems to present physical and "mental" retardation, perhaps due—among other things—to being under-fed. Symptoms are the following: major concentration difficulties, sudden behavioral changes (joy, sadness, stubbornness), frequent forms of agitation (stand up, walks on all fours in the classroom, hides under the tables, etc.). In addition, he is terrified of his father. Finally, he has eyesight problems, which to this day have not been taken care of by the family.

We would like your team to receive these students so that they can benefit from the advice of experts and consider the school and medical orientations best adapted to each of them.

The letter was signed by the high school's assistant principal, the chief education assistant, three teachers, an education counselor, and a nurse. As the letter was presented during MEDIACOR, it first triggered a short silence. We were all digesting the situations and details presented in the letter. This was followed by expressions of disbelief, particularly with respect to the "package" form this referral took. Reactions were split between those who felt that it was hostile and disrespectful to the students, that it brushed over certain complex situations, and that it readily pathologized behavior with very general information, and those who sensed that beneath this somewhat insensitive grouping of student portraits was an education team expressing its powerlessness in managing this challenging diversity of origins, educational levels, and social situations. After a long discussion, Dr. Bennegadi suggested we invite the education team to come meet with us, so we could have a better sense of how to help them.

A few weeks later, everyone except the assistant principal came to meet with us. They were all very eager to talk about their heavy stress load working in UPE2A classes. What came out of our discussion was that considering the conditions they worked under, their education mission could not be fulfilled, and in their respective functions, they all felt a deep sense of powerlessness. They were obviously emotionally caught up in the painful trajectories and precarious social situations many of their students were experiencing. They were critical of the lack of means provided to them by the state to carry out their jobs: there was no school psychologist, no social worker. One teacher I was seated next to confessed to the team that she felt at a loss with one of her students whom she had invited to stay with her. Now she felt uneasy managing a double role as teacher and host.

In responding to the particular situations of these students, Dr. Bennegadi gently called the team's attention to the issue of acculturative stress and its impact on students' learning and concentration capacities, which did not necessarily indicate the presence of cognitive or behavioral disorders. In fact, a major detail lacking from the referral letter was the students' time of arrival in France. After asking the professionals, we learned that all five students had arrived in France within the past year. Another important point was that none of the referred students had been to school in their country of origin. The team complained that they often received children with no formal status of "unaccompanied minor," and thus they did not benefit from any support from ASE—housing, most importantly. In addition, none of the students had received medical follow-up.

In response, MEDIACOR suggested that the students be referred to a Permanence d'accès aux soins de santé (PASS, Healthcare Access Platform)—a medical center where any checkup is free for a person aged sixteen or older—and advised the team to turn to the school physician to obtain state medical aid for them. We gave them the option of coming back to us if necessary, to address each child's situation. Therefore, without setting aside the potential relevance of psychological or psychiatric assessment or follow-up for some of these students, we helped to raise the consciousness of the professionals from the referring school to the structural constraints that shaped their problems: structural constraints of their own, because they were expected to fulfill a mission without institutional support, and structural determinants affecting the students' situation and related behavior. MEDIACOR team meetings, I would argue, are most critical in challenging the logics of an unfair system. Referring state agents, like the ones we received that day, often leave with a different interpretation of the situation than the one that initially motivated the referral. The question remains as to the impact this reconsideration has on them when they return to their institutional routine.

*   *   *

The study of school referrals encapsulates the various logics that were identified in chapter 3. On the one hand, it sheds light on how references to essentializing cultural representations rely on a local repertoire that makes interpretations of "suffering" readily definable and hence manageable. Specific representations of "migrant youth" as potentially dangerous delinquents, or stigmatizing discussions of "normal" behavior, affect how these children may be perceived in schools, as Murielle's comments illustrate. On the other hand, it highlights how the unfavorable structural conditions in which these children live are overlooked, not only because cultural interpretations come to the fore in explaining pathological behavior but also because a highly complex educational apparatus is deployed in assisting children with "difficulties." When referred to Centre Minkowska, such situations challenge transcultural professionals to deconstruct these social categories and the pathologizing processes at work while remaining attentive to the psychological impact of poorly negotiated hybrid identities for second-generation youth as well as destabilizing settlement conditions for recently arrived youth.

PART III ETHICAL DELIBERATIONS

As we have seen in part II, cultural difference is an easily mobilized rationale to legitimize referrals to specialized mental health institutions like Centre Minkowska. This culturalization of psychological distress and social ills leads specialized mental health professionals to experience the contradictions and double binds that derive from their identification by referring state agents as cultural experts. While these contradictions and double binds are anxiety producing, they also offer fertile ground for resistance and ethical response.

A critical analysis of the social situations in which migrants find themselves unveils how their vulnerable positionality within an unequal social order exposes them to psychological distress and potentially leads to disorders requiring clinical attention. The stakes of interpreting forms of "social suffering" and their origins are high for professionals at Centre Minkowska. How do we make sense of the overlapping of social determinants and individual distress? How can we avoid medicalizing or pathologizing the social while also allowing recognition of social determinants in caregiving practices?

The approach practiced at Centre Minkowska incorporates this critical stance through regular staff deliberations about how to engage referring professionals in considerations of the social roots of suffering in a psychotherapy context. In this last section, I first consider how professionals at Centre Minkowska have adapted their clinical practice to accommodate situations in which social issues are predominant and hinder psychotherapeutic work. I refer here to situations of extreme precarity, when patients' uncertainty about obtaining legal status or accessing basic needs (a place to sleep or food to eat) makes time chatting with a psychotherapist almost irrelevant. I then explore whether Centre Minkowska has been instrumentalized by the state as a stopgap for excluded migrant populations. In doing so, I investigate how ruptures between professionals' ideals and system logics fuel feelings of frustration and provide an impetus for staff members to take responsibility and action but also differentially affect experts according to their professional status and experience. Throughout, I highlight MEDIACOR meetings as opportunities to evaluate how Centre Minkowska professionals use the cultural competence approach.

5 · ENACTING CULTURAL COMPETENCE

When MEDIACOR was created in 2009, meetings took place for an hour once a week. Now they take place every day, Monday through Thursday. Much like the number of patients at Centre Minkowska, the number of referrals to MEDIACOR has increased steadily, from 189 referrals in 2012 to 1,083 in 2017. This represents an average of eight to ten referral letters a day. With only one person available to screen the letters—Audrey, occasionally assisted by Verthançia—and the involvement of the MEDIACOR team for the discussion of complex situations, it usually takes the center an average of two to three weeks to respond. In almost 90 percent of referral cases, PTSD is identified. About half of the referrals come from professionals within Paris; the rest are spread across surrounding areas. The highest share of referrals comes from the Seine-Saint-Denis department (93), directly north of Paris and characterized by a highly diverse and socioeconomically precarious population. The average age of referred individuals is thirty-three years old, and there is an almost even split between men and women. However, there are few family referrals (only 15 out of a total of 1,083). Twelve percent of referrals are for individuals under the age of eighteen (134 cases). Most referred individuals come from Afghanistan, Ivory Coast, Bangladesh, the Democratic Republic of Congo, Guinea-Conakry, Mali, Algeria, Sri Lanka, Nigeria, and Sudan.

Out of the total 1,083 referrals in 2017, 291 (27%) were redirected to sector-based clinics, associations, or other partner institutions. The remaining 792 patients were seen at the center, minimally for an evaluation session or a consultation at the clinic. Of the patients seen at the center, 142 necessitated the intervention of an interpreter. Close to half of all referrals came from social workers (250) and general practitioners (235). The remainder came from psychologists (110); social services assistants (103); special educators (89); psychiatrists (private or public) (87); hospital practitioners (all services) (85); school professionals (doctor, nurse, social worker, or teacher) (42); other medical or paramedical professionals (neurologist, midwife, occupational therapist) (26); legal professionals (lawyer, probation officer, judge) (23); social, family, and economy counselors (14); nurses (all sectors) (10); or volunteers and patients themselves (9).

From my experience, MEDIACOR has become a unique effective space for the transmission of knowledge about person-centered transcultural psychiatry and cultural competence; it is not a space for a typical staff meeting. Rather, it is designed to be formal but nonjudgmental. It is a space where therapists in training (TEFs) directly confront clinical situations and learn about complex referrals. "Therapists in training" is a term purposefully chosen over "interns" in MEDIACOR to reduce power asymmetries and encourage participation at the same level as clinical professionals. Staff members have developed a clinical case study sheet, which indicates important information TEFs need for understanding and presenting a case. This form, known as a *fiche de presentation*, was developed by MEDIACOR to help TEFs put the AMC (clinical medical anthropology) framework into practice.

The form has placeholders for basic demographic information TEFs are asked to collect in order to present a situation, which may be downloaded from the website and filled out by referring agents. Additionally, to improve the screening of referrals and to collect basic information needed for this process, staff also developed a referral form that duplicates this section of the form (see figure 1). The form then sketches additional areas of investigation, which follow the AMC model (see figure 2). The process of filling out the form enables TEFs to identify explanatory models of health as they appear in the referral—or, alternatively, to identify missing information.

Following the decision to base referrals on the AMC model, MEDIACOR established the form, with its own specific jargon, to lead staff and TEFs in presenting and analyzing clinical cases in a routine, formatted way. As TEFs present forms during MEDIACOR meetings, they are asked to address the three dimensions of the AMC model and to reference the areas about sickness (the individual's social situation), illness (the individual's interpretation of the situation), and disease (behavioral and somatic information, diagnosis). They use these words— "sickness," "illness," and "disease"—in English, as the creators of the AMC model wished. At the beginning of discussions, Dr. Bennegadi argued that there was no perfect translation for the words and that it was better to leave the concepts untranslated: in French, the word *maladie* encompasses these three notions, so it becomes problematic to translate them. This use of English was integrated into the center's everyday discourse to the point where some expressions circulate regularly, such as "Il a un *sickness* massif!" (There is a massive sickness) or "On sent que l'*illness* est prêt à émerger" (We can sense that the illness is ready to emerge). Meanwhile, the use of those terms strategically reinstates the theory underpinning them. Expertise, I suggest, often draws on such linguistic processes of socialization (continuous engagement with the objects of knowledge), authentication, authorization (the institution's active use of expertise to organize knowledge), and

Date: ....

Referring professional: ❏ Psychiatrist ❏ Psychologist ❏ Social worker
                         ❏ General practitioner ❏ Other (specify)

Address: ....
....

Referring institution:
❏ CADA (Asylum Seekers Housing Center)
❏ CHRS (Social housing)   ❏ ASE (Child Welfare Services)
❏ Healthcare institution   ❏ Legal institution
❏ School institution   ❏ Association

Address and telephone number: ....
....

Name of person referred : ....
Surname: ....
Address: ....
Tel: ....   Age: ....

Country of origin: ....

Date of arrival in France: ....

Language(s) spoken: ❏ French   ❏ Other languages (specify)
....

Family situation: ....

Administrative status: ❏ Asylum seeker   ❏ Migrant   ❏ Un-accompanied minor

                          ❏ Other (specify) ....

Immigration trajectory: ....

Asylum trajectory: ....

Elements of trauma: ❏ Yes   ❏ No
General practitioner: ❏ Yes   ❏ No
If so, contact information:
....
....

Somatic exploration(s)?   ❏ Yes   ❏ No
What kind? (attach results) ....

Medical treatment?   ❏ Yes   ❏ No
If so, what kind?:

Reason(s) for referral:
....
....
....
....

FIGURE 1. Basic Demographic Information and Form for Referring Agents

SICKNESS
Impact of social determinants on the patient's psychological state: ❏ Neutral ❏ Destabilizing
Impact of societal determinants on the patient's psychological state: ❏ Neutral ❏ Excluding ❏ Stigmatizing
Other contextual elements: ❏ Individual level ❏ Community level
ILLNESS
Does the patient express psychological distress via: Cultural representations from his/her cultural group: Linked to magical or religious values ❏ ❏ Unknown   Linked to spiritual values ❏ ❏ Unknown   Linked to traditional values ❏ ❏ Unknown
Cultural representations from the biopsychosocial model: Neuropsychiatric ❏ Psychological ❏ Psychoanalytical ❏   Systemic ❏ Sociopolitical ❏ Unknown ❏   Adult behavioral or personality disorder: Paranoid personality ❏ Schizoid personality ❏ Schizotypal personality ❏   Antisocial personality ❏ Borderline personality ❏ Histrionic personality ❏   Narcissistic personality ❏ Avoiding personality ❏ Dependent personality ❏   Obsessive compulsive personality ❏ Unknown ❏
Type of psychological defense mechanisms: Mature ❏ Immature ❏ Intermediary ❏ Unknown ❏
According to the elements of sickness, illness and personality, tentative diagnosis (DISEASE)   Therapeutic indications: ❏ Medical treatment ❏ Psychotherapy ❏ Sociotherapy

FIGURE 2. Categories of Information based on Clinical Medical Anthropology

naturalization (as expertise becomes familiar and integrated into clinical routine and language) (Ansari 2014). In other words, efforts to implement a new language to make sense of clinical situations not only reinforce the institution's unique identity but also transform participants' gazes: the organized categories of the *fiche de presentation* become a natural way of understanding participants' realities (Foucault [1963] 1994; Good and DelVecchio Good 1993). However, as

Dr. Bennegadi often reminds TEFs during meetings, the form is a didactic way of training people to gather information on important aspects of a health issue, but life itself is not always so neatly organized.

DECENTERING AND REFLEXIVITY

The outcome of the AMC model of organizing and interpreting information is that a person progressively becomes able to decenter from his or her own frame of cultural reference. This ability to decenter is an essential component of how we define "cultural competence" at Centre Minkowska.

MEDIACOR is a space where everyone is invited to cultivate this kind of reflexivity through being attentive to his or her own potential biases or projections. As Dr. Bennegadi often reminds us, "We all rely on stereotypes, but as professionals in the transcultural clinic, we have the responsibility to identify them, so as to not let them imbue our understanding of clinical situations. The stereotype self-imposes; the therapist disposes." Dr. Bennegadi insists that MEDIACOR meetings remain a safe space where divergence or disagreement may be freely expressed and where people with varying levels of clinical training have equal influence in discussions around and elucidation of referrals. Consider the following dialogue from a MEDIACOR meeting, which illustrates the values of decentering and reflexivity and the ways in which these meetings operate. Staff members are discussing the case of a fifty-year-old French citizen, born in Burkina Faso, who was referred to Minkowska by a psychologist because "he expresses his suffering on the register of superstitions and beliefs" (*il exprime sa souffrance sur le registre de supersititions et de croyances*):

TEF: Fifty-year-old man from Burkina, of French nationality, residing in [name of location].

DR. B: So he lives in Burkina or he was born in Burkina?

TEF: He was born in Burkina and arrived [in France] when he was fourteen. Now he is fifty.

DR. B: And so why is it not just indicated that he is a French national, before saying he comes from such or such country? There's no language issue. When he arrived he was fourteen. At fourteen, he learned French. So, let's keep on going and identify the potential slippages.

TEF: So it was not good to mention his origin and . . . ?

DR. B: No, that's just between us, to open the debate.

MJ: Although it simply says, Mr. X, born in Burkina on such date, of French nationality . . . it does not put forward . . .

DR. B: Yes, but when I describe you in order to refer you to Sainte Anne [a famous psychiatric hospital in Paris], I don't say, "She was born in Bordeaux of French nationality."

(*Several people laugh.*)

DR. B: I just say, "My colleague is doing poorly, would you please see her?"

MJ: But *I am a Bordeaux resident* before being French! (*Laughs.*) [emphasis hers]

DR. B: Well, nobody will penalize you for that. They will just say, "Ah, she comes from a place where they make good wine."

(*Everyone begins talking at the same time.*)

Here, Dr. Bennegadi draws attention to how individuals are presented and how identity is used. This recurrent exercise within MEDIACOR invites everyone to note how characteristics used by referring professionals to introduce individuals can affect others' perceptions of them—or even predispose us as clinicians to frame the individual in a certain way. In this case, the first sentence spoken by the TEF, if unexamined or probed further, might have characterized the man primarily in reference to his country of origin despite the fact that he had spent most of his life in France.

IDENTIFYING EXPLANATORY MODELS

After this debate about identity, the TEF continued his presentation and explained that the man had met his wife a decade after he arrived in France, and they now had four children, aged twelve through twenty-eight. In 2014, the family was evicted for not paying their rent and for a neighborhood disturbance:

TEF: In August 2015, they are referred to [an association] for temporary housing with social assistance.

DR. B: So, you mention all this so we are aware of the *sickness*—

TEF: Yes, the family's social situation.

DR. B: OK, so we don't know yet what happened to this family.

TEF: Is it too long?

DR. B: No, it's just that we know that he met this woman, although we don't know whether she comes from Burkina. . . . We can tell it's about a family who imploded, about a story related to debts, or something else . . . it hasn't been said yet.

TEF: So, the psychologist who wrote the referral mentions a serious psychological suffering. . . . Quickly, she mentions that the wife talks about recurring couple conflicts, each member of the couple feeling judged and rejected by the other. The husband reports he is the victim of a conspiracy.

DR. B: That's a nice start . . .

MJ: Yes, it [the referral] says that the wife is conniving with corrupted policemen.

DR. B: Ooh, that becomes complicated. . . . There are worrisome messages on the theme of conspiracy that this man sent to his social worker. In June, the association informs us that the wife left the house for another residence in [name of the town].

MJ: The social worker filed two reports.

DR. B: That's what is important to say; we must talk about the elements that intervene in the context of psychopathology. . . . [Are there] reports for violence from the husband on his wife?

MJ: It does not say.

TEF: Then there is a decision from Child Protection Services to place the youngest children . . . then there's something interesting: the husband refuses visits from his wife, saying he is the victim of sorcery and witchcraft (*maraboutage*).

DR. B: From policemen, too, or only from his wife?

TEF: No, only his wife. There are also somatic elements. It says that he has a follow-up at a medical center because he suffers from stroke sequelae and Type 1 diabetes. He takes medication[,] but there is no indication as to which ones. It adds that the patient agrees to be referred to a specialized institution, but at the same time, he is afraid that he will receive the confirmation that he is mad.

DR. B: Oh yeah, we can do that very well! (*Laughs.*)

For the first part of the referral analysis, Dr. Bennegadi allows the TEF to report on different aspects of the clinical situation as part of the AMC expert analytical process. In line with the AMC model, *sickness, illness,* and *disease* elements were brought together to try to construct a holistic understanding of the case. From this initial assessment, understood as comprehensive within the AMC model, staff members are then able to identify missing elements that are necessary to inform the referral decision—that is, to refer the patient elsewhere or to see him at the center. The consideration and synthesis of *sickness, illness,* and *disease* and the identification of missing elements constitute the knowledge basis of what staff members understand as "cultural competence," which is illustrated through the following dialogue:

DR. B: OK, bring out your competence now. Where is the cultural competence? First, what essential element do we need? The behavioral disorders we are being told about: did they exist before the stroke, or are they the consequence of the stroke? Because the stroke may cause behavioral disorders. Did he start mentioning sorcery before, or after? When he had his stroke, he went to the hospital, he took the treatment. His diabetes, I presume he takes his insulin, since it's Type 1 diabetes? If he doesn't take it, he dies. So, we need to clarify the organic and psychological circumstances to assess which one precedes the other. But we don't have that information. On the other hand, we know that the children suffered the consequences. So did the couple. . . . We also need to know the reason why they were evicted from their home: is it because of the noise from the fights, or is he the one who is paranoid in relation to those who assist the family? Here we're not just talking about cultural references, but social references as well. With the idea that "traditionally this is how we do [it] back home," when traditionally, things are different in France. Is it what started things, or not. . . . All of this provides us with information on his personality, so there is plenty of information missing, plenty. Who is asking for the referral?

MJ: The psychologist.

DR. B: What is her opinion on his behavior?

MJ: Great psychological suffering. She says he is depressed about the situation.

DR. B: This man surely has a doctor taking care of him. One cannot suffer a stroke, and not benefit from a follow-up. So, we need to get in touch with colleagues at the medical center. We need all this information so we may situate the *illness* discourse (*le discours de l'illness*) [emphasis his], . . . the cultural references to sorcery etc., in a context—if it's one way to put it because it's difficult to find the right words to talk about it, it has nothing to do with someone who is delirious. . . . It's not the same treatment. It's not the same approach.

Through this last part, Dr. Bennegadi emerges as orchestrating the discussion. Although he allows meeting participants to share their interpretations, he ensures that they return to the elements considered most relevant in the context of the AMC model. In this case, there are too many missing elements for MEDIACOR to make a decision, so Dr. Bennegadi invites the team to reflect again, as he did when the situation was introduced, on the ways representations of otherness potentially cloud our interpretation of situations:

DR. B: So, let me ask this provocative question. To what extent did it help us, or hinder us, to know that he was born in Burkina? If you can answer that question, it means that you did an enormous cleansing work against prejudices in your conscience. When we referred to a French citizen born in Burkina, what did it change in your mind? If I had introduced him as a Frenchman who married this woman and had children and then problems, diabetes etc., do you see him differently than when I say he was born in Burkina and he is French? Does it change his skin color, in your mind?

AUDREY (A) (NURSE): Well, when you say he comes from Burkina, evidently you don't see him as white!

DR. B: So, how do you imagine him to look?

A: Well, black!

DR. B: And why do you imagine him as black?

A: Because we were told he came from Burkina.

DR. B: See, that's all the work I've been trying to do here for a very long time by saying that I don't make a value judgment. It takes tremendous work on the way we look at the person, so as not to be oneself the victim of a reasoning that is useless, that may be problematic. It [that kind of reasoning] has to be secondary. It must not be pre- but rather post-person-centered. It's not that I don't see the color, but

I don't see the person *through* his color. That's not the same. That's not the same. It requires introspection. Then if we focus on skin color, we feel much more at ease to think about semiology. But if we start with skin color, we find ourselves with a prejudice, which is useless. It does not help me at all. From the same case, had you not mentioned Burkina, if you had mentioned another country, it would have changed things! The colleagues add this element because they discriminate involuntarily. [emphasis in the original]

Beyond attention brought to stigma and particularly to race, what Dr. Bennegadi invites professionals to practice is a kind of resistance to a priori forms of categorization when thinking about people. He thus calls for the same phenomenological attitude Eugène Minkowski attempted to formalize in his work: focusing first and foremost on the individual's experience of his or her disorder in a specific context.

DELIBERATING

This MEDIACOR vignette illustrates how the enactment of cultural competence relies on the process of deliberation. Commenting on the complexities of situations in PASS consultations, French social philosopher Marie Garrau (quoted in Georges-Tarragano, Girier-Debolt, and Davakan-Alonso 2017) highlights the value of deliberations in the health-care context: she notes that given the complexity and inherent singularity of each situation that professionals encounter, there cannot be a ready-made solution based on an existing rule. This means that "good" decisions are those that adapt to a particular situation under consideration. This requires professionals to use discernment and creativity. She also notes that a complex situation typically derives from heterogeneous elements. In that respect, deliberation involves responding to the complexity by acknowledging this in the first place. Her conclusion is based on three different arguments. First, deliberation enables the sharing of information and knowledge. Second, it combines temporal discussion with reflections on past experiences, constraints that weigh on present situations, and possibilities that may exist. Third, it constitutes the only available means for taking into account various points of view, as well as medical, ethical, and organizational demands, and integrating them in relation to a particular patient. In the end, successful deliberation requires a sense of collective action, humility, and attention from participants. In other words, it requires the capacity to distance oneself from the situation (Garrau, quoted in Georges-Tarragano, Girier-Debolt, and Davakan-Alonso 2017, 18; my translation).

In the many-factored complexities of the cases referred to Centre Minkowska, the practice of collective deliberation through MEDIACOR meetings helps illuminate multiple perspectives on any given situation. The meetings may help staff at the center redefine institutional responsibilities by enabling them to identify shortcomings or missing information. They teach professionals how to be flexible in the face of complex, multifaceted situations. As we will see in chapter 6, this deliberative framework may be tested when professionals feel strongly affected by situations of extreme suffering and injustice; they may experience a gap between their values of decentering and of reflexivity and the limits of the health system.

EMPATHY AND THE "SCHEMA OF SUFFERING"

A major outcome and an attribute of cultural competence, and of the ability to decenter in particular, is the capacity for a person to experience empathy in a context where cultural representations and moral values are likely to differ. According to referral narratives, state agents turned to Centre Minkowska partly because they felt lost in the face of such difference; they were unsure how to do more than they had already done. This is a typical issue we address in the context of professional training; for each patient or service user, professionals expect to be given a to-do list that is based on the person's cultural background. At the professional training department, Laetitia and Christine regularly encounter questions about whether they can tailor our cultural competence program to "Chinese mothers" or to "African families." It usually takes some negotiation over the telephone before such professionals, who request training, agree to let staff from the center first introduce the concept of decentering and then discuss more specific cultural representations through case studies. In the past decade, however, my experience with training professionals across health and social institutions has taught me that rather than the category of "culture," professionals increasingly struggle with the category of "migrant." The professionals I have encountered tend to view migrants as ultimate foreign subjects who, in the collective imaginary, trigger a hoard of signifiers (as seen in chapter 3). These signifiers impose various "schemas" of being, feeling, and acting that professionals expect to face when interacting with migrants.

In the context of an action-research project on mental health provision to non-French-speaking patients, funded by a French philanthropic network, I worked with the mental health team at a CMP in the spring of 2017.[1] I selected this CMP for participation because it frequently referred patients to Centre Minkowska on the basis of a "language barrier." One part of the research consisted in funding interpreter services for eighteen months in a selection of district CMPs and evaluated the outcome of this collaboration. The other part involved offering a three-day training session to participating teams on intercultural communication and techniques for working with interpreters in mental health care. The idea to organize this session came from our observations at MEDIACOR; a large and increasing number of referrals were coming from district CMPs and were motivated predominantly by the fact that the patients were non-French speaking.

On the last day of the training program at each CMP, we left room for the integration of theoretical and technical content through role playing and for the analysis of different situations that professionals might want to share. At one CMP, I co-led this session with a clinical psychologist and an anthropologist colleague, Daria Rostirolla. That morning, we asked if anyone wanted to share an experience from their practice, and a nurse volunteered to speak about a situation he had recently encountered for which he had needed a Tamil interpreter. When we do this kind of intervention, Daria follows a specific supervision framework that we ask everyone to respect: when a person first introduces a situation, only that person is allowed to speak. At the end of his or her presentation, we instruct the speaker to ask the whole team a specific question. In the second stage, team members are permitted to express their responses to the situation. Only at the end is the initial speaker allowed to react. That day, the nurse spoke about a twenty-five-year-old man from Afghanistan, who had to flee the country under unclear circumstances. On his asylum trajectory, which included the help of a *passeur* (smuggler), he had traveled through several countries but was finally stopped in Bulgaria, where he was beaten and tortured by the customs police and fingerprinted by authorities. Under the Dublin agreement, this meant that his asylum request had to be made in Bulgaria. He managed to leave the country, and a year later he arrived in France and submitted an asylum request, which was subsequently rejected. He then received a formal request from the government to leave the country.

The nurse, who was charged with taking down the stories of incoming patients at the CMP, then explained why he was bringing up this situation: "That man smiled all the way through the interview. I told myself, he left his family back home, his parents, he went through this difficult journey . . . how could he not be suffering? The others, they speak of atrocities. I wonder how one could know if someone has *really* suffered. . . . And there he is, making social demands. . . . Now I know that both are intertwined, I mean social circumstances here in France, and psychological suffering. But this man, he kept smiling" (emphasis mine).

When the nurse had finished summarizing the situation, my colleague asked him if he had a question. "My question," he said, "is how do we triage patients who have *real* needs[,] from a health care perspective, compared with those who only come with other interests?" (emphasis mine).

During the nurse's recitation of the situation, there had been palpable agitation in the room. Some people appeared to struggle to avoid expressing their irritation with their colleague. I heard one psychologist sitting near me mutter, "This is unbearable. I want to leave this room," as she nervously rolled a cigarette. As we opened up the discussion to the rest of the group, one psychologist gently addressed the nurse: "You know, we have to give ourselves the time to build a relationship with the person. It's not about a technique, it's about a relationship. That person's asylum trajectory and the tortures he mentioned are not just anecdotes. And someone who smiles is not necessarily someone who does not suffer. In fact, from a clinical perspective, it may lead us to identify a discordance."

At that point, a secretary commented on the nurse's observation, adding that migrants usually come with a "schema of suffering." She speculated that the reason her colleague was disturbed was because those common elements were absent: "The patient did not really play his part," she concluded.

Upon hearing the secretary's words, the psychologist who had earlier muttered his discontent interjected, "We are health care professionals! We listen to people! We don't police them! One has the right to ask for something else than care!"

Another psychologist, in a much calmer tone, continued, "Look, these people come from war-torn places. The journeys they go through, it's sheer horror, and you can't [always] read that on their faces."

The nurse responded, "Perhaps a more general question I have is how do we welcome people? What we do is not my definition of welcoming. We are intrusive; we may feel like we are policing people, even though we know we are just following protocols. . . . I mean, I think this raises the issue of the time we devote to welcoming people."

Another psychologist ended the discussion by saying, "We have to move beyond this suspicious positioning to create the conditions for a genuine encounter with the person, and we have to take distance from this practice of telling one's story. It may not always be culturally appropriate, just like that smile may have been."

From his clinical experience at the cultural consultation service in Montreal, transcultural psychiatrist Laurence Kirmayer (2008) wrote about the limits of empathy in the face of social difference. This issue has been explored by cultural anthropologists and ethnographers, and scholars have raised epistemological debates around the limits of cultural relativism. My own challenge as an ethnographer writing about "culture" is to maintain a level of reflexivity that enables me to move fluidly between the etic (the observer's point of view) and the emic (the point of view of the person observed). French phenomenologist Maurice Merleau-Ponty powerfully captured this uneasy equilibrium with the following question: "How can we understand the other without sacrificing her to our logics or without sacrificing her own?" ([1958] 2008; my translation).

In the ethnographic context, the anthropologist accesses the world of the persons she observes by living in it for a substantial amount of time. In the clinical setting, Kirmayer (2008) points out, the patient's lived world is not present and thus can only be imagined by the professional or investigated through questions. Among other barriers to empathy in an intercultural setting, Kirmayer identifies differences in verbal and nonverbal language and expressions; differences in life experiences; variations in cultural background knowledge, particularly in the domain of the implicit, understood as that which is unidentified because it is commonsensical or hidden because it is "embarrassing, secret, sacred or dangerous"); the social framing of the context of the encounter, "which includes extended family networks locally and abroad and the networks and institutions of the host society"; and the "strategic positions" (2008, 466) and goals of participants in the clinical encounter. The challenge to make sense of events in a transcultural consultation thus consists in "building up culturally plausible contexts and scenarios and asking the clinician to inhabit these scenarios, putting themselves in the patient's position" (Kirmayer 2008, 467–468).

In the vignette involving the nurse and the man from Afghanistan, for instance, the nurse's focus on the patient's smile was particularly salient; he considered its expression during a referral inappropriate, although it may have been motivated by the patient's psychological distress. As one psychologist noted, the smile may, clinically speaking, raise a red flag that signals discordance as a dissociative, schizophrenic symptom. Some members of the team expressed specific ideas about the social representation of the asylum seeker, such as when the secretary noted he did not exhibit the common symptoms of migrants' "schema of suffering." What appears crucially missing in this nurse's interpretation of the situation was recognition of any number of other possible motivators for the patient's smile. For instance, the asylum seeker might simply have been smiling out of politeness and deference in a setting that was necessarily asymmetric in terms of power dynamics. Another possibility was that from a cross-cultural perspective, smiling might indicate a wide variety of emotional states, such as self-control or an effort to hide negative feelings. What also appeared to affect the nurse's interpretation, which I routinely see in cases I come across in my own work, is the projection of his own life experience onto a patient. At the end of the discussion, the nurse spoke privately with me and explained that as a migrant from North Africa himself, he knew of the hardships of immigration, even though his was not traumatic—but he again reiterated that smiling was certainly not something he would expect of a recently arrived asylum seeker. In light of this information, I wondered whether the nurse was unconsciously projecting common social representations of North Africans onto the asylum seeker, such as the fact that North African migrants like himself are stigmatized in the media for being malingerers and profiteers of the system. Did he see the patient as a mirror image of himself?

While I have no way to answer this question definitively, since the nurse and I did not discuss it, the notions of cultural transference and countertransference are central to the cultural competence approach. In his seminal work *From Anxiety to Method in the Behavioral Sciences*, anthropologist and psychoanalyst George Devereux (1967) broadened the classic understanding of countertransference—defined by Freud as the result of the patient's influence on the clinician's unconscious feelings—by showing that what is experienced as radically different may produce anxiety. Relying on a psychoanalytic perspective and through detailed illustrations, Devereux (1967) argued that when confronted with phenomena or practices that appeared as transgressive in one's own culture, an observer might experience fascination and anxiety through the reactivation of repressed desires. He then identified the universal basis of what produces anxiety: anything that threatens the fundamental vulnerability of a human being; revives idiosyncratic anxieties related to the observer's personal history; and threatens to undermine the individual's main defenses, sublimations, and overall equilibrium. Devereux noted that in the face of such anxiety, any behavioral expert, such as an ethnographer, might resort to defense mechanisms that triggered distortions in the perception of the observed reality or subjects. These distortions may be related to the professional or sociocultural background of the observer, or to his age, gender, personality, beliefs, and so forth. In sum, Devereux noted that the observer will always attempt to interpret reality from his own cultural model of reference: to transform what is unknown into something that is known. In transcultural psychiatry, and more broadly in contemporary approaches to cultural competence, professionals are trained to be self-reflexive and to identify processes of cultural transference and countertransference, so they do not negatively influence the clinical relationship (Rouchon et al. 2009).

As illustrated in the vignettes about the nurse and Dr. Duriez's interactions with the Kouyate family in chapter 3, some of the professionals who work in the mental health field with migrants categorically expressed negative countertransference. Moreover, in my experience, the country's general climate of suspicion and repression, related to the social representations of migrants I identified in chapter 1, led to some of these professionals' negative countertransference during encounters with migrants. This climate affected professionals who felt the need to identify and differentiate between migrants who showed "real" distress and those who instrumentalized not only health care but welfare services in general (Fassin and d'Halluin 2005; Larchanché 2012; Ticktin 2011). This in turn affected professionals' health-care ethics and their capacity to relate to "the migrant" as a socially constructed category.

AN ATTEMPT TO REESTABLISH EMPATHY IN MEDIACOR

In the field of migrant mental health, a wide variety of state agents confront what they consider extreme social difference, as illustrated in the example recounted by the nurse. At Centre Minkowska, staff regularly noted that agents' motives for referral are affected by processes of negative countertransference, feelings of anxiety about the unknown, and feeling overwhelmed by situations they felt unable to handle. One referral that demonstrated these motivations particularly comes to mind. The letter, written by a special educator from the ASE, recounted the situation of Mrs. Ndongo, a single mother from Cameroon who had experienced trouble becoming pregnant but who eventually had two daughters, Victoria and Hope (aged ten and six, respectively). She had come to France with her mother as a little girl, and they had intended to join her father, who had migrated a few years earlier. The referral letter presented her as being the couple's only child. Mrs. Ndongo told ASE professionals that having an only child had been her parents' desire, as it served witchcraft purposes, and her parents always wished to do her wrong and prevent her from ever being happy. She also shared that, as a child, she saw her father have sexual intercourse with her in the world of spirits. She noted that when she told her mother about it, her mother did not react.

According to Mrs. Ndongo, she had married a man from Cameroon in her early twenties, but her father deemed the relationship doomed. She then recounted details about the couple's failed attempts to have children, spiritual ceremonies that were organized in Cameroon to figure out why she was not becoming pregnant, and the family's conclusion that her inability to have children resulted from the fact that she was married to her father in the world of spirits. The letter noted that it was this that led to her first divorce, but it offered few details about the circumstances of her meeting the father of her older daughter, Victoria, except that what precipitated their separation was Victoria's revelation to her mother that she had had sexual intercourse with her father in the world of spirits. Victoria also reported to her that in that world, she was a siren, had lots of sexual intercourse, and was a very tall mother of ten children.

At the time of the referral, the woman was no longer in contact with either of her daughters' fathers. The special educator then explained that Mrs. Ndongo had asked for Victoria and Hope to be placed in foster care because they had revealed their intention to kill her. The special educator reported that the girls confirmed this scenario to ASE professionals and said they had tried to kill their mother with a knife once and to weaken her by poisoning a chicken. Victoria and Hope explained that their maternal grandparents told them to do this—in their heads—and that unless they followed the instructions, they would die. The girls said that they needed to kill people, so that they could eat their spirits and gain more power. The special educator said she worried about the girls' situation but also about their mother, who seemed isolated in her attempts to protect herself from the influence of anyone else. The ASE team contacted a cultural association that would help them better understand what exactly was happening, but Mrs. Ndongo reportedly refused, saying she no longer trusted people—especially those of her own culture. Regardless, she respected and understood the team's need for advice on the situation.

The MEDIACOR team accepted this referral, and we decided to see Victoria and Hope first and to pay particular attention to how they interacted with each other and with the rest of the team. We asked the girls to draw, which they did for the whole session. As they drew, we first asked questions about school and then about who the older girl plays with and how she takes care of her younger sister. They both interacted easily with us and even seemed to enjoy the attention. At some point, Dr. Bennegadi even said to us, "Beware, I see you are all seduced right now! Let's re-center." The interaction between the two sisters was striking, and we could all see that their bond was strong. We asked a few questions about their mother, and at the end, Verthançia suggested they draw a picture to symbolize their relationship with her. Dr. Bennegadi was careful not to directly reference or investigate their mother's accusations from the referral letter: "There's no point in testing them on their mother's projections. Our goal today and main objective was to evaluate whether the girls are doing well, and if there is anything more we can do to help this family. Obviously, they have a healthy relationship between themselves, and with their host family. Let's not unsettle anything at this point."

We then offered to see Mrs. Ndongo. We were unsure whether she would accept, since the referral letter reported she was defensive with other professionals who cared for her daughters and limited contact to a minimum. To our surprise, she accepted. When Mrs. Ndongo saw us at the appointment, she told us that she had decided to come because she had been told that we were people open to alternative ways of understanding reality; she felt the center might be a space where she would not be judged. She came to a MEDIACOR meeting and did not seem intimidated by the group in any way. She was poised and direct, and spoke with quiet sophistication. She introduced herself as the executive assistant of an important firm, and we sensed her self-portrayal was meant to convince us to take her seriously. As she explained, "I'm not sure why I came. You have to understand that I gave my daughters away because I had to, not because I don't love them. I love them very much. I did what I did to save my own life." Dr. Bennegadi promptly asked her whether she would tell us a few things about the situation and how her daughters were threatening her.

In response, Mrs. Ndongo recounted the following event: "It was a beautiful summer day. The window was open and outside there was a wedding celebration, a Turkish one I believe. People were dressed beautifully, with beautiful colors. The married couple seemed so happy. I turned to the girls and asked them: 'Wouldn't it be nice if mommy found a boyfriend, got married, and we would be a happy family like that?' But they looked at me and in unison answered a simple but unequivocal 'No!' See, this is exactly what I mean." She then continued to recount how the girls would leave amulets under her bed meant to call a spirit, or tell her they were such and such princess or spirit that would come to take her life. Her allegations drastically contrasted with the behavior we witnessed from her daughters. When Mrs. Ndongo said, "I know you think this is nonsense, but it is real," Marie Jo reassured her that we were not judging her beliefs, and that she was familiar with such beliefs from having helped patients from the same cultural region.

"Let us help you," Dr. Bennegadi said. "We respect what you believe in. We are not going to tell you any other way. But we have our own way of understanding the situation and of possibly helping you solve it. That would mean that you would be willing to come back here and speak with a therapist, with Marie-Jo for example."

This approach and the group's positive, open attitude seemed to create the possibility for a therapeutic alliance. As Mrs. Ndongo left the room, she agreed to call back for an appointment with Marie-Jo. A week later, however, the special educator who had accompanied Victoria and Hope at the first meeting informed us that this would be unlikely to happen. One of the girls' psychologists had, probably unintentionally, characterized Mrs. Ndongo's cultural references as "fantasies." During a mediated meeting with their mother, the girls repeated what the psychologist had said. Furious, the woman left, threatening that they would never hear from her again. She never called or returned to the center.

*   *   *

The cultural competence approach at Centre Minkowska refers to the ability to identify explanatory models of health, disease, and healing—as they are defined in medical anthropology theory—and to resist a priori forms of categorization when interacting with migrants. In the context of mental health, cultural competence partly refers to understanding patients' cultural representations about suffering and about how to alleviate it. However, the term also refers to understanding mental health professionals' own cultural representations when they interpret patients' suffering and when they speak of the wide spectrum of social and societal determinants that trigger psychological distress or negatively affect it. This involves recognizing the structures that shape clinical interactions and rearticulating the cultural formulations of referrals in structural terms (Metzl and Hansen 2018, 115). In that respect, cultural competence first and foremost relies on professionals' ability to be reflexive and thus to decenter from their own frames of reference. The capacity to decenter is a work of posture, based on reflexivity and distanciation, with which anthropologists are familiar. It is challenging to acquire since identifying and questioning one's frame of reference is not a comfortable exercise, to say the least. It requires a person to acknowledge his or her own prejudices and to accept the necessity of occupying a position of not knowing; however, both actions are antithetical to common definitions of expertise and competence in most professional realms.

The cultural competence approach is most visibly enacted during MEDIACOR meetings through the practice of deliberation, which fosters pluridisciplinarity in exchanges. The meetings also position cultural competence as a sense-making framework rather than a normative practice. In chapter 6, we will see how important this deliberative space becomes when transcultural professionals' ideals are confronted with the violence of structural inequalities and the challenges of addressing the systemic needs of their patients.

6 · PSYCHOTHERAPY AT THE BORDERLAND

I startle as Mrs. Siaka loudly and repeatedly pounds her fist on the desk that separates us in the consultation room. She screams at me: "Stop saying that! Stop saying things are going to be okay. Things are not going to be okay. I have been struggling every day for the past few years, and things have been getting worse. I am tired. Look, my body is giving up on me. I am tired. I want to be there for my children tomorrow. I want them to remember me as a strong woman, as a mother who supported them."

Mrs. Siaka came to France from Cameroon in 2012. She traveled alone, pregnant with her fifth child. Back home, she was a busy, independent woman who trained as an athlete and worked as a coach. She even participated in national competitions. During one consultation, she told me her husband would often complain that she was too busy; she even spent some weekends away from home, when she participated in tournaments with her team, although she took her children along.

Mrs. Siaka was born to a Christian family, but her husband was born Muslim. They had a daughter born out of wedlock, and for some time they lived with Mrs. Siaka's parents. Mr. Siaka then decided to convert to Christianity, after which the couple married and later moved to Yaounde. Mr. Siaka's conversion created tensions between Mrs. Siaka and her in-laws, who were convinced that Mrs. Siaka and her parents had pressured him to convert. The couple had two more children, a boy born in 2002 and a girl in 2005. When Mrs. Siaka became pregnant with her fourth child, her in-laws started pressuring her to have her daughters undergo genital cutting. She vehemently opposed this, and as the pressure grew stronger, Mrs. Siaka fled to her parents' home. For a while her husband visited her and the children on a regular basis, but he failed to convince her to go back with him. To make ends meet, Mrs. Siaka began to trade clothing with neighboring Nigeria. At the end of 2011, during one of her trips, she met a man, James, a clothes supplier, with whom she had an affair. She became pregnant and attempted to get a medical abortion but failed. Her parents insisted that she keep the child.

One late afternoon in the summer of 2012, as Mrs. Siaka and her family were attending mass, the lights went out and shooting started from the back of the church. (Mrs. Siaka believes the shooters were members of the jihadist group, Boko Haram.) Most churchgoers died that day. Mrs. Siaka was spared by one of the shooters who recognized her (they had attended university together) and realized she was pregnant. She escaped and hid in the bush. With the little money she had, she took a bus to Lagos, hoping to find James, but she heard from one of his friends, Francis, that he had left for France. When she called her family, she learned that her parents were dead and that her children were missing. (She would learn a year later that her children had survived and been placed in a boarding school in Yaounde.) She stayed in Lagos for about a month. Francis helped her obtain a fake passport, and she took a plane to Paris in the early fall of 2012.

On arriving in France, Mrs. Siaka looked for James but never found him. A month later, she gave birth to a healthy baby girl. Two months later, Mrs. Siaka was hit by a car as she crossed the street while pushing a stroller with her baby daughter. Her daughter was uninjured, but Mrs. Siaka's arm was severely injured, and she lost the use of it. At that point she had not applied for asylum. For almost a year she had no residence permit and had to ask friends for money to pay for physical therapy sessions, but she became unable to follow-up with the necessary treatment, which delayed her recovery. She became very depressed, even after she obtained asylum-seeker status, which allowed her to access universal health coverage and to see rehabilitation specialists.

Ultimately, her asylum request was rejected, but she was granted a one-year renewable visa for medical reasons. When I last saw her in 2017, the *préfecture*, for reasons unknown, had failed to deliver her renewal visa. Instead, she was granted a three-month *récepissé* (residence permit), which allows her to maintain legal status but prevents her from receiving welfare benefits. She is therefore a legal resident of France with housing provided, but she can barely afford food and clothing. In one of our early meetings, Mrs. Siaka told me she could cope with such material struggles if only she could keep busy doing something. Instead, she said she stays home alone with nothing on which to focus but her continuous bodily pain. She cried over her feelings of powerlessness. I contacted her social worker to assess whether Mrs. Siaka could volunteer at a local NGO. Mrs. Siaka resides in a region that has far fewer opportunities for NGO activity than does Paris, but the social worker still managed to obtain an interview for Mrs. Siaka. Unfortunately, the woman at the NGO who received them held Mrs. Siaka in contempt; she told her to face the fact that her disability and limited French would likely make it impossible for her to get a volunteer position anywhere. Mrs. Siaka was devastated.

On this day, I feel I am partly responsible for Mrs. Siaka's reactive outburst. In the face of her despair, I feel a sense of helplessness and briefly stepped out of my position as a psychotherapist. I feel the futility of psychotherapeutic work at this particular moment: the accumulation of many different factors, from social to structural, have hindered Mrs. Siaka's ability to live the life she wants and continually challenge what she understands as the purpose of her existence. In this moment, I relate to the way state agents—social workers in particular—often feel baffled at their inability to support clients in situations like Mrs. Siaka's. On another level, I realize that she has come to Centre Minkowska, in despair and on edge, as a last resort.

*   *   *

Structural vulnerability, such as that which Mrs. Siaka faces, engenders suffering. State agents who refer people like Mrs. Siaka to Centre Minkowska do not always do so using rationales that psychopathologize patients. Some refer patients who, they realize, are suffering after repeated state failures along national social support pathways. However, structural vulnerability is often challenging to address, particularly by individuals at state institutions. Hence, many refer patients with these kinds of problems to a specialized mental health center like Minkowska, where structural vulnerability is routinely considered within the systemic approach underpinning the clinical medical anthropology model.

However, therapeutic consideration of structural vulnerability crucially requires that patients be willing to think reflexively about their lives in relation to larger social structures. Clinicians at Centre Minkowska regularly acknowledge that patients may not be immediately ready to engage in this kind of introspection. As a result, center staff assume a kind of vulnerable position of their own: they accept that part or most of their work will involve what is internally called "psychosocial support." This is a form of clinical listening that occurs without the patient engaging in the introspection necessary for what staff members consider a successful therapeutic encounter. But there is an inherent risk in assuming the role of therapist as only a clinical listener: people may simply offer an outlet for listening or compassion—without any kind of critical reflection on a situation—and in doing so normalize or even trivialize forms of social suffering (Fassin 2006).

In this context, critical questions around the role of therapists arise. Are we, as therapists, merely participating in appeasing the emotional burden of intolerable situations? Should we caution against and speak out about unfair social orders? Or should we compromise and operate from a position of critical pragmatism? As a medical anthropologist, I am aware of the effects of social structures on different forms of suffering, but I am also caught in the messiness of institutional work. This positionality causes me to struggle often with these questions. In this chapter, I address the logics behind and consequences of using Centre Minkowska as an institutional stopgap for situations faced by migrants that are primarily structural in origin. The center has become, over time, a stopgap that is not temporary but is relied on systematically by social agents from other institutions. In doing so, it has become a *borderland institution*. Here, I explore the structural logics that undergird this evolution. I argue that this is related to the disinvestment of the state in mental health care, and the types of liminal spaces—in all aspects of social life—that have been created as a result.

THE SOCIAL PRODUCTION OF SUFFERING

Liminal Lives

Our global economy and its forms of governance have progressively increased the number of displaced people living in different kinds of liminal situations, such as Mrs. Siaka. Rather than referring to them as "immigrants," "refugees," or "asylum seekers," Michel Agier (2013, 2016) proposes an alternative terminology: *hommes/femmes-frontières* (border men/women). This enables us to avoid the political narrative to which migrants are subjected and to depict their situation from a decentered, anthropological standpoint. The condition of these border men/women, Agier tells us, is characterized by long—at times indefinite—periods of time lived in situations of in-betweenness or liminality. The very locations in which they live may be characterized as liminal: camps, transit zones, borders. Agier uses different theoretical figures for these border dwellers to better apprehend their lived experience: the *wanderer*, the *métèque*, and the *pariah*.

The wanderers are those who roam around the Mediterranean or European points of entry through deserts, seaports, and streets. Their trajectories and destinations are often uncertain. They temporarily gather in makeshift camps. Agier notes that although ideas about the figure of the wanderer have a long history in western Europe as elsewhere, there are ever more of them in contemporary times. The *métèque* is another figure with a long history. In ancient Greece, the term referred to those who contributed economically to the city through their labor but enjoyed no legal or property rights because they were socially undesirable. Contemporary *métèques* are undocumented workers whose presence is now commonplace in urban centers or intensive agricultural landscapes. They stay in underground locations, such as squats, or they rent insalubrious rooms from unscrupulous landlords. Finally, pariahs are those who live reclusively in camps, as refugees, displaced persons, or detainees. They are stuck at the city edges, negotiating a new form of social life that is shared with individuals all over the world.

All three of the figures Agier proposes get by in life by using new ways of being in the world, with more or less ease and economic or social success. The unstable or transitory nature of borderland states or locations is not necessarily synonymous with anomie. In fact, at the center, we see alternative forms of sociality and cultural or political relatedness that emerge in patient narratives and allow them to be resilient. However, we also see that such borderland situations produce structural vulnerability. Over time, added to preexisting traumatic experiences related to migrants' reasons for migration, borderland situations have the capacity to take a toll on migrants' psychological well-being. Migrants' resilience is particularly tested by experiences of waiting in conditions of uncertainty, precariousness, adversity, and fear—as Mrs. Siaka's story illustrates. Such situations place individuals in a state of "existential limbo" (Haas 2017; Sargent and Larchanché-Kim 2006), which at best produce extreme fatigue and anxiety, and at worse, severe mental illness and risks of self-harm or other forms of violence.

Inhospitable Housing

Housing is central in analyzing how public policies affect migrant populations and how they produce anxious situations for migrants and for social or health professionals attending to their needs. Labor migrants have long been the object of specific housing policies in *foyers* (hostels), located at the periphery of urban centers and managed by a housing company called SONACOTRA (Société nationale de construction de logements pour les travailleurs). With the end of labor migration and the introduction of restrictive immigration policies, public authorities sought to see these *foyers* disappear and combined them with other "social housing" structures (e.g., for single young workers or the elderly), which became sites for marginalized or excluded populations (Bernardot 2008). In 2006, SONACOTRA became ADOMA (from the latin *ad* meaning "toward," and *domus* meaning "home"), and the company expanded to include emergency and temporary housing for asylum seekers, which were known as Centre d'accueil des demandeurs d'asile (CADA). In 1995, ADOMA managed five CADAs. Today, it manages 192 buildings, with 7,168 beds—25 percent of the total National Housing System (DNA, Dispositif national d'accueil).

The number of asylum requests in France has increased steadily since 2014, from over 65,000 requests that year to almost 86,000 in 2016 (OFPRA 2018)—and the trend continues. This upswing in demand over a short period of time led to saturation in the DNA housing structures. Housing and Orientation Centers (CAOs, Centres d'accueil et d'orientation) were created in 2015 to offer temporary housing to asylum seekers evacuated from overcrowded camps, but these do not constitute a long-term alternative for stable housing. Unless asylum seekers find community associations or close relatives or friends able to house them, they often find themselves on the streets. Over the past few years, the government's Office for the Protection of Refugees and Stateless Persons, known as OFPRA, has granted international protection and refugee status to an increasing number of asylum seekers, but the latter still find themselves without housing.

The professionals who work at CADA and other housing centers do so with limited means. These centers operate within a competitive system based on proposal calls for funding—a system that militant associations and social actors working with migrants have criticized as a commodification of social aid. The centers are evaluated based on their capacity to justify their actions and reduce costs. The cost–benefit rationale underlying the logic of housing funding affects the quality of social and health services and mental health services in particular. Although housing agencies employed their own psychologists in the past, many have had to cut these positions and rely on external services due to funding shortages. Over the course of only a few years, the ratio of staff members to residents at CADAs has shifted from one staff member for ten residents, to one staff member for fifteen residents today (Zeroug-Vial, Couriol, and Chambon 2014, 4). Likewise, the provision of social services within CADAs is extremely limited and is worse for emergency housing units, which have even fewer resources and professionals. Paradoxically, emergency housing seems costlier for both state and local budgets than does housing in more stable centers, such as CADAs (Zeroug-Vial, Couriol, and Chambon 2014). Therefore, the government's unwillingness to increase the number of CADA centers as a strategy to regulate migration and to reduce related costs is an illusory cost-saving mechanism, since unstable housing costs more than stable housing.

In its report on vulnerable populations' access to rights and health care in France, the NGO Médecins du monde (2016) indicates that among the asylum seekers received by Centres d'accueil de soins et d'orientation (CASOs, health and orientation screening and referral centers for vulnerable and socially excluded populations), one-third live on the streets, and only 18 percent live in housing provided by an organization or association. While the organization acknowledges that efforts have been made to increase the housing capacity of CADAs, it also reports a continuing decline in welcoming conditions for asylum seekers. The report notes that among adult foreign nationals, 68 percent are undocumented, and 24 percent are in a precarious administrative situation with less than six-month visas or temporary visas. In the context of medical and social service visits at CASOs, more than a third of undocumented people declared that they limit travel for fear of being arrested.

Asylum and immigration have both been the objects of recent reform. The first reform occurred in 2015 and sought to speed up the processing of asylum requests, build housing centers across the region, and reduce the delay in recording asylum requests to three days. Once a request is recorded, the asylum seeker is given a temporary residence authorization, which is renewed until a final decision is made by the National Court for Asylum Seekers (CNDA, Cour nationale du droit d'asile). There are two processing regimes: normal, which takes five months and involves a three-judge final examination at the CNDA, and accelerated, which takes five weeks and uses a one-judge final examination at the CNDA. A second round of reform law was passed in 2016, and its objectives were to fight the precarious conditions of migrants' residence in France by providing multiyear visas rather than visas for one year, six months, or one month at a time. The law also ensured that undocumented migrants and those whose asylum requests had been rejected were quickly deported to their countries of origin.

Following the 2011 landmark ruling of the European Court of Human Rights in the *M.S.S. vs. Belgium and Greece* case,[1] the notion of "vulnerability" was introduced into European legislation on asylum to encourage authorities to arrange special procedural guarantees for vulnerable people, such as unaccompanied minors; people with disabilities; people who had been subject to human trafficking; or people who had experienced torture, rape, or other forms of psychological, physical, or sexual violence. In France, evaluations of such vulnerability are carried out by agents of the French Office for Immigration and Integration (OFII, Office Français de l'immigration et de l'intégration); they are the first people to interview migrants during asylum applications. Because this evaluation interview occurs immediately upon migrants' entry into France, is relatively short, and is limited to "objective" and visible vulnerabilities through the October 23, 2015, decree,[2] French asylum legislation from 2015 allows for other vulnerabilities to be detected during later stages of the asylum process. CADA professionals are thus tasked with identifying and evaluating migrants' vulnerabilities. However, they are not provided specific guidelines or training to carry out this mission, which makes it difficult for such vulnerabilities (particularly psychological ones) to be properly considered. Moreover, asylum seekers who cannot benefit from housing due to the lack of available space receive only the initial OFII evaluation, and any specific needs they may have, regardless of "objective" vulnerabilities, are not taken into account. In short, without new guidelines and tools, legal procedures and housing conditions will continue to overlook critical vulnerabilities in migrant populations, which may not readily appear during the initial OFII interview.

The majority of asylum seekers are denied asylum. In 2016, 28.8 percent of asylum seekers received protection from OFPRA, and an additional 10 percent received protection in appeal from CNDA (OFPRA 2018). These figures vary according to nationality. For example, nearly all Syrian asylum seekers received protection from OFPRA in 2016 (OFPRA 2018). Among those rejected, most remain in France but without documentation and thus without access to state services. Some may be protected from deportation if they prove they have been exposed to death threats in their home country. Health care and legal trajectories for these populations often intertwine, particularly when requests for asylum are rejected and people are encouraged to apply for a residence permit for medical reasons. However, when such permits are granted, only a one-year stay is granted, although the permit can be renewed if the individual's state of health has not improved. Mental health is frequently invoked in such applications, since individuals may legitimately claim trauma experienced in their home countries following violence and persecution, linked to life circumstances in France, or related to situations of extreme insecurity and poverty.

Health Care and the Politics of Deservingness and Scarcity

In the face of such adverse social conditions and related suffering, how is the health-care system responding? In 2016, following an investigation of health-care refusals, the National Rights Advocate identified two physicians who refused to see patients with universal health coverage (CMU), which is the primary form of insurance for people not otherwise covered by employers, private insurance, or state medical aid (AME), which is health coverage provided by the state for undocumented residents. In January 2017, three different associations referred to the same National Rights Advocate a website that rejected CMU beneficiaries for online appointments.[3] In response, a health-care law was passed in January 2016 that created a commission to investigate and report on health-care refusals. The study and report commissioned by the National Rights Advocate, published in March 2017, highlight the impact of negative social representations on physicians and dentists about "the CMUs," which are considered to be "demanding" while "cost[ing] . . . a lot of money" (Desprès and Lombrail 2017, 5).[4]

On the topics of AME or the "waiting allowance," some media outlets regularly denounce the weight of this aid on the national budget or on the burden to French taxpayers. In the 2010s, the AME budget was the object of multiple Parliament debates in direct relation to immigration, despite the fact that immigration policies partly caused the increasing number of AME applicants and beneficiaries. While AME-related expenses constitute a mere 0.4 percent of the overall social security budget, these political debates have led to three different general audits, all of which "unanimously minimized the weight of fraud and pleaded in favor of maintaining the benefit" (Izambert 2016, 99).

Given the national turn in public health administration toward rationing health care on the basis of cost–benefit analyses rather than on the needs of patients, as explained in chapters 1 and 2, a culture has been fostered in which decisions have to be made about who deserves care and who does not. What Izambert (2016) calls *a staging of scarcity* legitimates practices of triage, even though they are at odds with health-care professional's moral values. In other words, it has been left up to individual health-care professionals to decide who deserves care and who does not. This is an ethical quandary people have to navigate every day.

"Precarious" Migrants and Psychiatry: A French Paradox

French sociologists Nicolas Chambon and Gwen Le Goff (2016) note that in the name of universalism and health-care access for all, no specific references to migrants or foreigners are made in mental health texts or reports addressing vulnerable publics. The 2011–2015 *Plan psychiatrie et santé mentale* (Psychiatry and mental health plan) (Ministère des Solidarités et de la Santé, 2012) refers only to "health care access inequalities." Language is the only identified obstacle to health-care access, while medical, social, and administrative aspects are ignored. The authors refer to the Robiliard (2013) report on mental health and the future of psychiatry, which highlights that the poor and asylum seekers fall outside the national sectorization system, which collates individuals' proof of residence by sector and acts as an administrative basis for many state institutions. Substitute domicile documents, such as an "administrative domiciliation"—an address created for those who are homeless or who have temporary housing so they may receive mail—are not always accepted by public, sector-based psychiatric institutions like CMPs. The Robiliard report refers to those who fall outside sectorization as "the forgotten" or "non-francophone" populations whose healthcare access should therefore be "adapted"—in other words, psychiatrists should address linguistic and cultural differences. The author of the report adds that "the concepts developed, among others, by Dr. Tobie Nathan . . . in relation to ethnopsychiatry, can be of great utility in the health care context for this part of the population" (Robiliard 2013, 34).

A controversy exists in France between those who defend universal health-care access and those who vouch for specific health-care platforms that are mainly managed by civil society through associations. Patients who remain in mainstream health care are directed to PASS clinics, some of which are specifically dedicated to psychiatry. While migrants comprise a large majority of PASS patients, clinic budget constraints often limit the use of interpreters, consequently limiting the provision of health care to these populations. Among obstacles to individuals' mental well-being, the most recent Health Ministry Report on mental health (Laforcade 2016) mentions constrained migration, lack of health-care access, extreme poverty, political forms of violence, and human rights violations. The report thus alerted policy makers that mental health prevention and intervention programs cannot be limited to the psychiatric treatment of mental disorders and must take into consideration social and structural factors. Nonetheless, while asylum seekers are identified in the 2016 report as a particularly vulnerable public, the government did not act on this information: no structures were created to specifically address the mental health needs of migrants for fear of challenging republican ideals about universal health-care access (Rechtman 2012). Migrants thus remain associated with "vulnerable" and "excluded" populations and benefit from mainstream institutions specifically dedicated to precarious populations, such as PASS clinics, Mobile Psychiatry for Precarity Teams (EMPP, Equipes mobiles psychiatrie précarité), and CASOs run by Médecins de monde.

Clinicians at these institutions, however, are not always trained to handle the specific health needs of migrants who have accumulated trauma and other vulnerabilities linked to their social environment. The recent emergence of certain clinical paradigms, such as the *clinical approach to exile* (Benslama 2004) or the *clinic of trauma* (Baubet et al. 2004), indicate the need for new clinical and therapeutic modes of intervention. When interacting with government-deemed "vulnerable" migrants, clinicians and other professionals are often put in positions where they must question their traditional caregiving practices. In the clinical context in particular, this entails acknowledging migrants' humanity and the contexts of rupture, loss, and dehumanizing precariousness many have endured. French sociologist Nicolas Chambon (2013) explains that mental health professionals may feel that they are being asked to manage situations that reach far beyond their skills and tasked with solving social as well as medical issues. For these professionals, beyond offering a space for psychotherapy, clinics like Centre Minkowska represent a place of hospitality and stability.

In these circumstances, the challenge is to maintain the meaning of caregiving. This challenge is exacerbated by work with a population for whom the meaning of psychotherapy, including its logics, duration, and regularity, is far from evident. Many clinicians at Centre Minkowska thus regularly face instances when patients do not come to appointments or arrive late. The reasons for these missed or late appointments vary. Sometimes they are related to structural constraints, such as lack of money to pay for transportation, and sometimes the stigma of being referred to a psychiatry clinic immediately triggers fears of being labeled "mad." Other times, the migrants' reasons are simply unknown to clinicians. In other words, a thorough understanding of migrants' situations sometimes escapes the health-care professionals who attempt to work with them, leading to migrants being perceived as "overwhelming" (*une figure du débordement*) (Chambon 2013). Professionals who work with migrants often feel overwhelmed; the complexity of the migrants' situations challenges the classical frame of professionals' mission and training to provide care. As a result, they refer migrant patients to specialized clinics like Centre Minkowska.

Referral of an Overwhelming Figure

The following patient was referred to us from a social worker at a CADA in a distant city in southern France. This is unusual, but Centre Minkowska is not affiliated with any one sector, so it may technically receive referrals or see patients from anywhere in France. The social worker downloaded and completed the referral sheet from the center's website but included no references to cultural representations. That day, the form was presented by Audrey, the center's nurse. As I mentioned earlier, Audrey is the last team member to have joined the center, right after completing her nursing studies. Out of all the center's full- and part-time staff members, she is the most private person. Although she eats lunch at the office almost every day, she rarely shares coffee breaks when everyone gathers together in the morning or after lunch. She is in her mid-twenties, and her young age sometimes makes it difficult for her to manage the medical secretaries, who are older and consider themselves to be more experienced than she is. However, the work she has done since being hired in 2016 is much appreciated; she has made a real difference in the way we process and triage incoming referrals, which is now being done in a much more efficient and speedy manner.

Audrey introduced the situation of Hamza, a twenty-four-year-old man from Afghanistan who spoke only Dari and who had arrived in France in the summer of 2016. We knew few details of Hamza's life story. We did know, however, that when he arrived in Paris, he was taken care of by a French NGO that manages CADAs and was immediately transferred to the CADA where he currently resides.

His father, a member of the Taliban, had been killed by the government's police. Hamza had apparently begun to feel that his family was being persecuted by the Afghani government and the police. He described these circumstances in his asylum request, and his social worker was concerned that this would be problematic regarding OFPRA's decision.

In the referral letter, the social worker reported that a few months after Hamza's arrival, she and her colleagues had visited the apartment he was staying in and discovered that it was quite dilapidated. Attached to the referral were photographs of the apartment showing holes in the doors and walls, which seemed as though they had been punched multiple times. Some walls were broken from floor to ceiling, and a radiator looked as though it had been pulled from the wall: twisted plumbing and broken pipes were skewed haphazardly away from their support.

Audrey continued to summarize the situation. At his request, Hamza was driven to the district emergency psychiatric service, where he saw a psychiatrist who prescribed an antidepressant treatment. According to the social worker, Hamza may not have taken the treatment, but he saw the psychiatrist twice. Despite this, he continued to damage the walls, as the photographs showed. At the beginning, they were holes, but the walls ended up being completely destroyed. There were also problems with the neighbors, and complaints against him were filed by ADOMA (the public housing manager). In response, a hospitalization request was made by a judge. Hamza was admitted to the same hospital by the same psychiatrist, who thought Hamza could leave the hospital because he did not think Hamza suffered from a psychiatric pathology; rather, he thought it was "merely" a behavioral disorder. He held this opinion even though Hamza had been hospitalized under constraint. The psychiatrist decided to let Hamza go at the end of the day. Again, the social worker realized that Hamza never took the prescribed treatment—the antidepressant and the anxiety medication—and that he had continued to damage the apartment. This time, he had destroyed the plumbing installation. Ultimately, ADOMA filed a new complaint.

Earlier that day, Audrey had called the social worker to get more information. The social worker informed her that for the past few months, they had received more complaints, including from the local police, who reported that Hamza has assaulted people in the street and damaged "things" outside. As a result, ADOMA was planning to "let go" of him by requesting that he be transferred to the Paris area, with the condition that he receive medical follow-up in the CADA where he was being transferred. The social worker complained to Audrey that the local psychiatric hospital had not done anything for Hamza, and that the local CMP did not want to see him with an interpreter either. At that point, Verthançia, who had also been in touch with Hamza's social worker, added that Hamza himself reported feeling threatened when he was in the street, and that he was extremely anxious about his asylum request. "In any case," concluded Marie-Jo, "they are waiting for our advice, and we told them that our institution is not able to deal with the situation." Audrey reiterated that in the South of France, where there is little infrastructure catering to migrants specifically, including interpreter services, CADA professionals feel helpless in the face of such situations. To this comment, Dr. Cheref reacted with what I interpreted as mild irritation:

DR. C: What do you mean they don't have anything? They have a psychiatric service.

A: Yes, but . . .

V: Before mailing us this referral letter, the social worker called us last week. I'm the one who spoke with her, and it's true that they are completely helpless. . . . For example, she explains that the CMP won't see him with an interpreter. They raise the financial issue.

DR. C: They are helpless? In the psychiatry service, I count one, two, three, four, five, six psychiatrists.

We debated why, in the face of such a serious situation, the associated health professionals did not mobilize, and particularly why they resisted using an interpreter. Given Hamza's history and social situation, there seemed to be a dramatic disconnect between health professionals' medical conclusions and the observations of other professionals associated with him, supported by photographic evidence. We all wondered: How do we make sense of such a complex situation and respond appropriately to the referral from a holistic perspective—that is, from a perspective that takes into consideration individual, institutional, and societal dimensions?

What follows illustrates the deliberations that typically take place during MEDIACOR. Staff members strive to produce a comprehensive approach to each situation, which may then enable a pragmatic response from a more distanced perspective. Deliberations like these involve confrontation between broad ethical principles, which staff members identify in relation to a situation—illustrated here by references to medical ideas about the nature of duty and obligation, the evaluations carried out by psychiatrists based on "objective" diagnostic categories, and the legal frame of constrained care—and the personal ethics of referring professionals and MEDIACOR participants. Through the following exchanges, the didactic component of MEDIACOR meetings—the implementation of a cultural competence approach—is also illustrated. Here I deliberately include the data in dialogue format to illustrate the back-and-forth exchanges between staff members and the tensions that arose from this.

DR. B: Okay, I suggest we take advantage of the situation, of this *skandalon* (scandal), so as to discuss how the health care system functions, so that people understand how it works, how it is district based, how there are people and institutions for that, the police, psychiatrists. . . . Now, the issue is well framed. To this issue that was raised, I would like three answers. The first is the psychiatric issue, and I will ask Dr. Cheref to summarize the situation. The second is the social issue. I would like Verthançia to give her opinion. And the third is institutional, and I will ask Marie-Jo to respond. This is an instructive case, let's go. Dr. Cheref, can you please let us know what the law and the profession . . .

DR. C: The law doesn't . . . it just looks at the behavioral disorder. The behavioral disorder is a symptom. The person has to be hospitalized, under such conditions, to evaluate the nature of the behavioral disorder, what does the behavioral disorder mean, period. . . . In my opinion, personally, he was evaluated once, no, twice, once by one psychiatrist and once by another, both from the same district, and I would personally not try to suggest any idea about a diagnosis when they have had the patient in front of them, [and] they established he had behavioral disorders. As far as I'm concerned, from here, I would not allow myself to say it is this, or it is that, especially since in my opinion, this will end up becoming a legal case. . . . The hospitalization under constraint was not maintained following a consultation with the hospital's psychiatrist. So, a psychiatrist saw the individual and deemed that his state was not compatible with a hospitalization under constraint.

DR. B: Was he released with a treatment, do they say that?

A: No! Well yes, with [an antidepressant] and [an anxiolytic], but he didn't take them.

DR. B: So, hear the arguments well. These are professional arguments, not some moody arguments. Colleagues have seen him and have estimated he's not delusional. They fulfilled their responsibility. Okay? And not one said anything different. . . . So, people did their job, and the response is: behavioral disorder. Okay. You have photographs, images, people who say he breaks everything, etc., that he's aggressive, that's another matter. Now, the social dimension. We have one part of the elements. Now we're going to see about the global situation. We cannot lecture people on that. So, what is the social dimension? Let's limit ourselves to the *sickness*. What's the social dimension? What issues does this raise for us? For our own personal ethics? What's going on there?

DR. C: I would add a point here. We are not even called on by the psychiatry staff, who don't ask for anything. We are called on as a psychiatry support unit by social workers so that they can explain to us the attitude of health care professionals towards one of their residents.

In the first part of the interpretation of this situation by staff members, the medical elements are identified and debated. Dr. Cheref defends the positions of the outside health-care professionals, concluding that from an objective, clinical standpoint, "a psychiatrist saw the individual and deemed that his state was not compatible with a hospitalization under constraint." From his perspective, the only response the center should give the referring social worker is the same: no other action is necessary on a medical basis. Dr. B, however, pushes the conversation toward other considerations:

DR. B: [We've heard the medical considerations, but] MEDIACOR is organized in such a way that we can consider the social. So, you hear the arguments made by Dr. Cheref. The medical part took responsibility for its arguments. Now let's talk about something else. The floor goes to Verthançia. And Audrey, if you have things to add, you add them. It's that [social] dimension for the moment.

V: I was talking about the CADA. I find they have a lot of goodwill, but in such a situation, they could put a person out on the street, without ensuring housing follow-up. They have no obligation. And as I said, I talked to the social worker, and I can really tell she's in an uncomfortable situation, because she says, "I see a man suffering a great deal, and I am very limited."

DR. B: How is she limited? Tell us.

V: She is limited in the sense that for her, this is a purely medical issue, with respect to what she witnesses there daily, and the behavior he displays, but that when she tries . . .

DR. B: Okay, then stop here, stop here. What is the first question we may ask ourselves? About what we just heard?

TEF: Why does she see those disorders when the psychiatrists don't?

DR. B: Yes, but the psychiatrists, we were told that they evaluated him, and they gave an opinion. What is the most commonsense position from a professional point of view? I work in the CADA, I worry, I see this behavior, I do everything necessary, the police take him to the hospital, the psychiatrists say he can't be hospitalized under constraint, because it would be a violation to the individual's freedom—there are laws for that in France. They prescribe him an antidepressant and an anxiolytic, which means they think he's not even psychotic, and that all he does is because he is very anxious in light of his history and his trauma. We're okay with that. Now, the person who contacted Verthançia, what does she need to do? Again?

V: I suggested she call the CMP professionals again. I really suggested that she insist, that she request to speak with the person in charge, to the head doctor . . .

DR. B: Exactly, and tell them the situation. She has the perfect right to do so. . . . We give her advice so that she is able to question the local doctors: "I called a team who knows about these issues, here's what they think." For us, it is clear that our colleagues should see him again and confirm what they reported. Are these only behavioral disorders, or something else? And we can emphasize that the presence of an interpreter seems to be of utmost importance to improve communication, etc. There, that's it. *There's nothing else we can do. It's out of the question for us to engage and do the work for someone else. First of all, that's not our role, and second, it would completely miss the point. We are not the ones who should act.* (my emphasis)

In this second part of the MEDIACOR deliberations, which broaden the perspective to take into account social and institutional dynamics, staff members directly engaged with the referring social worker's experience, both through the testimonies of MEDIACOR professionals who interacted with her—Verthançia and

Audrey—and through Dr. Bennegadi's situational reasoning, in which he imagines what the social worker might say: "I work in the CADA, I worry, I see this behavior, I do everything necessary. " The situation is no longer detached from the context, as it was at the beginning of deliberations, when it was presented through a medical interpretive frame. Despite the fact that this particular situation falls outside the boundaries of the center's outpatient care, MEDIACOR's mission is to craft a follow-up response that provides the referring professional with a concrete proposition for what to do: in this case, staff at the center suggested that the social worker encourage the patient's health professionals to reevaluate him in the presence of an interpreter.

In this particular instance, deliberations also helped redefine institutional responsibilities. The conclusion of staff members' deliberation was that there was no room or reason for Centre Minkowska to accept the referral or do anything other than affirm the social worker's concerns and identify options for the general improvement of clinical evaluation practices and related caregiving—namely, suggesting the intervention of a professional interpreter. However, Dr. Bennegadi's concluding comments about how it is "out of the question" for the center's staff to "engage and do the work for someone else" indicates his sense of irritation with the reasoning behind the request. It also expresses his weariness at the overall absurdity of the situation: that for a man in such an obvious state of despair, no mainstream institutional support could be found.

ACTING AS A STOPGAP: CONSEQUENCES AND RESPONSES

A central question this situation raises is this: Does Centre Minkowska, despite its status as a state public health institution but with the humanist ethos of its community-based roots, function unofficially as a humanitarian organization? Does it act as both mediator and stopgap for mental health services that migrant populations need? The center occupies a unique position. Unlike humanitarian NGOs, it works within the confines of the state. And yet its position at the borderland created by intersecting institutions leads it to face the same tensions as NGOs—namely to risk maintaining the status quo on migrants' unequal treatment and to keep discriminatory practices invisible. To some extent, the center's unique expertise in caring for those who are excluded from other mainstream institutions may indirectly encourage referring state institutions to remain exclusionary—those institutions will see no need to expand their mandates because they have an alternative on which they can rely. This sometimes raises ethical dilemmas and outright feelings of frustration when staff members encounter referrals for which the referring agents cannot or will not engage with migrant patients themselves and instead prefer to abdicate responsibility to someone else. MEDIACOR helps mediate such reactions by staff members.

The Affective Logics of Work

How do staff members react to referrals like the one just described? Audrey provides a strong example. Other than a three-month internship in the pediatric unit of a major Parisian hospital, she had had no formal professional experience before working at Centre Minkowska. She had never heard of the center before applying to fill the medical secretary position—a temporary position she chose while waiting for a job opening as a nurse in another medical institution. However, her application was timely. Following the second round of HAS certification, inspectors had penalized the center for not meeting patients' basic physical examination standards; as a result, the center's evaluation score for the pain-management category of the evaluation was significantly lower. Staff members considered what to do and decided they should hire a nurse. Audrey was looking for a position in psychiatry because she was concerned about her work environment and did not want a technical position in another hospital service. During a conversation with her about her reasons for joining the center, she explained:

> Besides the center's activity, I appreciated its institutional dynamics. I liked how professionals communicated and how relations seemed healthy and calm. It is nice to go to work and know that your colleagues are nice. . . . That would be very rare in a hospital setting, at least where nurses work. I was interested in the MEDIACOR, the work on patients' referrals. And finally, the encounter with patients, their life trajectories, the issue of immigration and asylum . . . it is a timely issue and it is very interesting. . . . I didn't know anything about it, but it interested me, and I easily integrated into this place. I felt like I was going to feel comfortable here.

Considering her lack of work experience, it is unlikely that she would have been given the same responsibilities elsewhere as she now has as the coordinator of MEDIACOR. With the help of the medical secretaries she supervises, Audrey filters incoming referrals and contacts referring professionals for additional information or to direct patients to other services. She is conscientious about her job and regularly stays after hours to finish paperwork. Given her commitment to the center, strong caregiving ethics, and relatively recent experience within the health-care system, Audrey regularly encounters situations that challenge her moral ideals and lead to indignation in the face of professional disengagement.

Following deliberations around Hamza's violent behavior, Dr. Bennegadi dictated the response we should send to the social worker. Various jokes followed, and the tense atmosphere dissipated. "See how the situation affects you," Dr. Bennegadi commented, "the fact that we are not helping someone who is doing badly (we were in an altered state). . . . MEDIACOR is in a trance!" He then asked if anyone wanted to comment on the decision or on how they felt about the negotiation.

A: Again, it seems to me extremely serious, this issue of medical responsibility.

DR. B (*in a soft but firm tone*): Audrey, you have no grounds to stand up in any way and in any manner against medical responsibility. You don't know anything. You don't know what happened. So, you cannot generalize that way . . .

A: It's the hospital, it's not normal!

DR. B: Maybe, but from what MEDIACOR can observe from Paris . . . well, I would add that this mail would be even more efficient if Verthançia could call the person back to tell her, "We discussed the situation, we wrote you a letter that can help you, do not hesitate to use it to question colleagues." That's it. We did the job. We don't abandon colleagues when they ask for help.

MJ: OK, let's move on to the rest of the *fiches*.

DR. B: Hold on, because I can see that Audrey's still angry.

A: It's not anger, it's not . . .

DR. B: Come on, you can unload. You were moved by this situation.

A: Well, it's not that I'm moved . . . It's always the same problem. I'm the one who opens the mail, and it's a recurring problem. And in this case, it's very serious. As far as I'm concerned, if someone I know tomorrow is assaulted by this person, do I agree with the psychiatrist's position? I mean, you can't protect them. . . . I know that in my position as a simple nurse, I couldn't say he certainly made a mistake, and perhaps he didn't make any, but considering the photographs, I think there is a problem, that Hamza is not doing well, I think. And I may be mistaken, perhaps the doctor is right. In fact, I think it's because the patient could not speak French, and that he [the doctor] surely said, "Oh no, I don't know," and he preferred getting rid of the situation. But in this case, there are complaints.

DR. B: You raised an issue of concern to the field of mental health everywhere, and particularly here in France, about the limits and about the freedom of the patient and the mentally ill. The laws of 1848 and 1870 insist that we do not rely on impressions to hospitalize someone. So, it's important that you understand this is a societal debate, not a debate between individuals.

Audrey's comments convey her sense of frustration in the face of referring institutions that take advantage of Centre Minkowska's services and of these institutions' related disengagement. In usual MEDIACOR settings, Dr. Bennegadi encourages the expression of affect, not to expose the person but to foster reflexivity. In this session in particular, however, I also had the sense that Dr. Bennegadi, as a physician, felt ill at ease with the question of medical responsibility (as did Dr. Cheref earlier on). During deliberations, he seemed particularly eager to vouch for his colleagues, even making assumptions about how seriously they had taken their responsibility. As Audrey continued to voice her doubts over the medical evaluation of Hamza's behavior, he chose to question the social worker's responsibility instead:

DR. B: Well, she [the social worker] can call too; let her take her responsibility, as well, and call them. Tell them there is a risk, so they know about it.

A: But they know about it; they filed a complaint.

DR. B: Well, if more elements are brought to their attention, if the social worker shares her anxiety of the risks by bringing more information, the shrink will see things differently! He's not going to screw up. He can't. He is responsible for the patient's health! Maybe he was just told, "Oh, it's a refugee. He has issues." We can help fill out the information, so the colleagues realize that there may be something. They must do the job of informing and insisting, by relying on the mail. That's the public health role we play. That's how we are efficient.

MEDIACOR thus offers a space where affect can be expressed and, to some extent, legitimately participate in the logics of professional deliberation itself. In this conversation, Audrey, a young nurse, downplays the weight of her own arguments in the face of medical decisions when she says, "In my position as a simple nurse, I couldn't say he certainly made a mistake, and perhaps he didn't make any." However, with Dr. Bennegadi's encouragement, she finds a way to articulate her ethical reasoning and express her sense of discomfort. Dr. Bennegadi responds to each of her comments from an institutional perspective, tentatively reasserting the reasons behind Centre Minkowska's decision not to intervene directly. This kind of "affective deliberation" offers staff members the possibility of considering other perspectives and decentering their own biases—as the following shows:

DR. B (to Audrey): You are in the B phase of people who work at Minkowska. Phase A is fascination. Phase B is indignation. And the third phase, coming up, will be . . . decentering and cultural competence. You have no choice. You cannot . . . if you didn't care about it, you wouldn't talk about it. Since you care about it, and since what we discuss here touches upon what is human, and sometimes it is unbearable, it's very good that we can manage the emotional within the technical. We are alive. We don't see this problem from a distance. It moves us. So, we must be able to be moved while we keep decentering. It's important. But it's normal. It's a normal process. Verthançia went through this, and she can tell you about it. We almost hospitalized her, almost!

(Laughs.)

Beneath the protective functions of humor and metaphor, Audrey and Dr. Bennegadi question the legitimacy of the action required by Centre Minkowska in this case, and safely express their ambivalence about the motives of referring state professionals. The cultural competence approach advocated by the center supports the expression and consideration of many different perspectives among staff members. It also provides a deliberative framework through which people's emotions, feelings, and ideas—in relation to their everyday work—can be discussed and managed. This allows staff members to learn how to cope with the limits of the health system in which they must—necessarily—work. Decentering—or the ability to adopt a more distanced, objective viewpoint—and the management of affective logics of work (the capacity to work through people's emotions, feelings, and ideas) are thus integrated into the cultural competence approach. Decentering, in this framework, does not entail condoning discriminatory referrals or violent situations, such as the one exposed here. Rather, it is an asset that allows professionals to deal with complex situations on a daily basis, a work of posture that defines the very possibility of managing uncertainty and of accepting situations in which a person is in a position of "not-knowing" (Guzder and Rousseau 2013). I would argue that this capacity for professionals to express their empathy and humanity, as Dr. Bennegadi himself underscored, may be particularly productive in the face of situations of suffering and injustice.

The ideas proposed by MEDIACOR about notions of duty and obligation, and the cultural competence framework at Centre Minkowska more broadly, contrast with the traditional professional deontologies that require people to repress or control emotions. In their ethnography of another borderland institution—a "mobile psychiatry of precarity unit"—anthropologists Aline Sarrandon-Eck and Cyril Farnarier show how emotions can be involved and how they play out in decision-making processes, "at times playing as important a role as medical rationality . . . as professionals directly advocate for an urgent situation concerning a person who particularly affected them" (2014, 176). While the practice of decentering may not directly subvert an unfair system that produces the violent situations professionals from Centre Minkowska encounter, it provides humane and healthy interstices of action and caregiving that nourish the possibility of finding meaning in one's work and therefore the energy to take action.

THE DIFFERENTIAL IMPACT OF AFFECT AND AGENCY

Another dimension appears from the deliberations in this particular MEDIACOR case: not all professionals are equal in negotiating affect and in achieving a sense of agency in their work at Centre Minkowska. As I mentioned earlier, despite MEDIACOR's goal to promote symmetry in professional exchanges and to make such exchanges a safe space for the expression of affect, Audrey is quite clearly limited in her ability to defend her argument that medical responsibility may be at stake in this particular situation. This, I argue, is likely related to her age, gender, and professional status. In fact, I admit that I sometimes find Dr. Bennegadi's skills in leading and orchestrating MEDIACOR meetings a bit patronizing and paternalistic. Such limitations to the ideals and values promoted by MEDIACOR through its cultural competence framework emerge in other

professional settings at the center as well. In the remainder of this chapter, I analyze how, depending on their professional statuses and missions, Minkowska
professionals' negotiations of affect and agency are likely to differ.

Vouching for Migrants' Legitimacy

Beyond structurally complex situations for which Centre Minkowska acts as a pal-
liative stopgap for larger systemic dysfunction, there are specific referrals for
patients who need help establishing the legitimacy of their illness for asylum purposes. In these instances, migrants who provide proof of psychological or psychiatric follow-up at a mental health institution like Centre Minkowska sometimes
garner compassion from those who judge their situations. Miriam Ticktin (2011)
skillfully documents how migrants use the illness clause in France and how bureau-
crats and other state officials translate claims about human suffering into state
recognition. In doing so, she observes that state agents reinforce a regime of care
in which the suffering body is the only morally legitimate way for migrants to
access state rights, including residence status. She shows that what state agents
uphold as a humanitarian acknowledgment of the universal biological body—and
a moral mandate to protect its integrity beyond the dictates of politics—functions
in practice as a way to reproduce inequalities on the basis of racial, gendered, and
geopolitical hierarchies.

In a recent analysis, d'Halluin-Mabillot (2012) shows how debates about
deservingness emerge even among institutions that support asylum seekers. This
leads to different ethical stances: some argue that questions about deservingness interfere with the therapeutic mission of health professionals, while others
acknowledge that health-sanctioned asylum applications cannot be discounted
precisely because they constitute an extra chance at asylum. The following vignette
about Mrs. Diallo, a woman from Guinea, illustrates how such debates unfold at
Centre Minkowska.

Mrs. Diallo escaped persecution in Guinea in 2015. Her older daughter underwent genital cutting against her parents' consent and died a few days later as a consequence of hemorrhage. To protect her two younger daughters and recently
born son, she decided to flee. Her husband organized their trip to France but
stayed behind for financial reasons. He has been forced to hide from relatives for
fear of retaliation. During the MEDIACOR evaluation of Mrs. Diallo's case, we
identified trauma symptoms (sleep disorder characterized by vivid nightmares,
chest pains, and a state of hypervigilance). She also expressed suicidal thoughts.
Our colleague, Dr. Carlin, was scheduled to see her but was absent the day she
arrived. We arranged for emergency treatment through another psychiatrist, who
gave her an antidepressant and an anxiolytic. We debated scheduling a follow-
up for her at Centre Minkowska, but she was housed in a CADA in a distant
city, which was a three-hour train ride from Paris. According to her social worker,
the local CMP was unable to offer follow-up in English and refused to call an

interpreter. Mrs. Diallo had a general practitioner who had agreed to assist with her treatment but could not provide psychotherapy.

The follow-up certificate, written by Dr. Carlin, states that Mrs. Diallo lives in a state of constant anxiety and hypervigilance, which is exacerbated by sleep disorders, nightmares, and headaches. She was diagnosed with PTSD (F43.1) and general anxiety (F41.1) (the diagnosis codes are based on the International Classification of Diseases, ICD-10). In the end, we decided to see Mrs. Diallo at the center on a monthly basis. Her CADA was paying for her train tickets to Paris. Although her symptoms had not improved, she was able to get more sleep with the help of the medication. However, her asylum request was rejected by OFPRA, which caused more anxiety, and she appealed to CNDA. At the center consultation following her court hearing, she was utterly distressed. Before she said anything to me, she handed over an envelope. In it, a letter from her lawyer stated concerns about Mrs. Diallo's behavior during the court session and how it may have been interpreted by the judges. First, she said Mrs. Diallo's story about her family's asylum motives and journey was somewhat incoherent. Apparently, she had named some dates and key players in a different order than what appeared in the official narrative. Second, Mrs. Diallo had appeared emotionless, and her lawyer was concerned that such a lack of affect may have raised judges' suspicions about the veracity of her testimony.

The lawyer then asked Dr. Carlin to produce two new medical certificates. The first certificate, she said, should support Mrs. Diallo. She asked whether Mrs. Diallo's medication could possibly have "annihilated emotions," which would explain why she appeared emotionless in court, "even when referring to the atrocities she experienced." She also asked whether the medication or trauma itself could interfere with her memory or understanding of time and space. If so, the lawyer intimated, this could explain why Mrs. Diallo had "inverted both the dates and people present" when she recounted two events that had happened close to her daughter's death. The second request was for Dr. Carlin to conduct a psychiatric evaluation of Mrs. Diallo's daughters "because you know their story. It will certainly not be easy out of one evaluation to ascertain their state of mind, but your contribution would be valuable. Do they have fear associated with their history? Do they fear going back to Guinea? Are they conscious of what happened to their sister? How do they feel about it? Are they sad to see their mother in such psychological distress? Sad not to see their father or to have regular news from him?" The objective of the certificates was to dispel any doubts judges may have had about Mrs. Diallo's story and to support the necessity of granting protection to Mrs. Diallo's daughters.

As I read the letter and talked with Mrs. Diallo, I felt increasingly irritated with the administrative aspects of the situation. Mrs. Diallo told me that her lawyer had scolded her after the court session, and I was outraged. In addition to the stress Mrs. Diallo experienced because of testifying in court, she was overwhelmed with guilt for having "failed" the CNDA interview. Her daughters were present in court, witnessed the lawyer's tactless reprimand, and were anxious about the outcome of the session. They have had nightmares ever since. Finally, upon returning home, the CADA director called Mrs. Diallo to the office and prepared her for what would happen if her request was rejected by CNDA. She told Mrs. Diallo that the government was taking increased measures to circumvent illegal immigration and that expulsion practices would be enforced.

Dr. Carlin's reaction was calmer than mine. As I shared my response with her, she said she had adopted a militant position on the issue of certificates. She had work experience in the humanitarian field, both with Médecins sans frontières and Médecins du monde, and explained that in the context of health-care provision to vulnerable populations, she considered issuing such certificates an extension of her work as a psychiatrist. Specifically, it aligned with addressing the social context of her patients: "As long as it is a process shared by the patient within the boundaries of confidentiality, and to the extent that it is faithful to the clinical situation, I find no problem in the use of certificates in legal procedures." She underscored that working at a place like Centre Minkowska supported her personal commitment to care for all who experience trauma—whether related to immigration or not: "It may seem very strong a word, but to me this is a vocation." She explained that when she began volunteering at Médecins du monde in Spain with so-called "economic immigrants," she began to question the underlying dynamics of migration and exile:

> I felt I could be useful in providing support to people experiencing extreme suffering, who had been victims of torture, rape, or war . . . and I came to practice this kind of support directly in the field through humanitarian action, mainly in Palestinian territory where I stayed for a long time, but also during an exploratory mission in Morocco with immigrants who are stuck there in transit zones . . . and so in that sense it is vocational because I told myself, that type of support is really hard, but someone has to do it, and as far as I'm concerned, I can relate to it, it has a special echo in me. . . . It also relates to my activism, which I was unable to carry through in the context of humanitarian work for personal reasons; I could not see myself change my life or places every two years. On the other hand, I felt like something would stop abruptly for me if I did not pursue work in that context. Obviously, there is a lot of precarity, of injustice, but this is at the limits, at the frontier. Because it is political. A lot of those who come for asylum, who end up being rejected, most of these people could easily find a job and make a new life for themselves. So, the fact of being able to accompany and to care for what, according to me, initially does not have to become pathological, it was linked to this mission. I strongly felt that way.

In the thesis she wrote for a continuing education program in psychopathology and psychotrauma, in which she relates her experience working at Centre

Minkowska with asylum seekers, Carlin (2017) explains that she found herself trapped in a maternal role within the therapeutic context—a place where the only support she could provide was listening to asylum seekers. In situations in which her cases lacked a dedicated social worker, she let practical issues enter the therapeutic space and often found herself playing the role of a "therapist of the social." She wrote: "For a long time, I felt little legitimacy with respect to my professional skill, because I had overreached my expected role; but on the other hand, I felt that no psychological progress would be possible for these patients if social necessities were not dealt with *at the minimum*" (2017, 28; my translation, emphasis in original). According to Carlin, the challenge of caring for asylum seekers is preserving the therapeutic space from external factors while also dealing with the particular demands and time constraints imposed by institutional administration (2017, 31). Dr. Carlin's positioning, I suggest, offers a nuanced counterpoint to Miriam Ticktin's (2011) argument that participating in the logics of compassion inevitably causes the kind of unfair order these logics attempt to subvert, by way of hiding structural inequalities and indirectly reproducing them. I argue that therapists' acts of social buttressing within the health-care relationship itself constitutes a form of political engagement; therapists like Dr. Carlin support individuals who would otherwise find themselves in an institutional wasteland—unable to gain support from professionals within mainstream health structures and unable to locate other forms of help at the fringes of the formal sector. In this way, social support and caregiving relations can be political. Instead of a relationship that reduces individuals to stereotypes of legitimate suffering victims, therapists like Dr. Carlin provide migrants with the means of existing as both complex and singular human beings.

Engaging with Futility

In relation to finding forms of agency through professional positions, Verthançia's experience as a social worker contrasts with Dr. Carlin's experience as a psychiatrist. Headed to work one morning, I crossed paths with Verthançia. We live in the same suburb and often meet in the metro on our way to work. As a social-work student, she was interested in the impact of cultural representations on the practice of social work, especially situations in which the social worker and client share the same cultural background. She noted, "I ended up not choosing this topic [for research], as I was told this was too polemic a subject." But she remained curious about how migrants negotiated different systems of care, particularly in the field of mental health. At first, she had even wanted to become a psychologist, and working at Centre Minkowska seemed an ideal place.

In her current work, Verthançia said she measures how important it is for professionals to understand the basics of mental disorders: "There are so many gaps, so many situations in which people act out and we could have avoided it." She expressed dismay at the amount of bias she had seen affect professionals' referrals and found herself "peeved" or "disconcerted" when she observed that "attitudes don't evolve." Verthançia is a bold and assertive woman, but as a social worker, she is often exposed to situations of extreme precarity and vulnerability. While clinicians at the center offer psychological support to migrants, people tend to expect Verthançia to come up with concrete solutions to their problems—especially those related to emergency housing, health-care coverage applications, and administrative status.

That morning, Verthançia ruminated over something that had occurred the day before. She had received a young woman who had been "Dublined": her fingerprints had been taken in Italy. Since it was the country through which she first entered Europe, the Dublin agreement mandated that she apply for asylum there, and she had received a letter from the prefecture stating that she must return to the border so her asylum request could be processed. The woman saw Marie-Jo first but was referred to Verthançia for assessment about what could be done at an administrative level to appeal the decision. Verthançia had never met the woman and had no information regarding her trajectory, so she said she could not directly write a support letter for her. Instead, she referred her to a legal association where she could speak with volunteer lawyers and noted that in any case, a letter from a social worker would not have much weight.

Verthançia now told me the story of what followed: "I am still shocked at what happened yesterday. Right after our meeting, this woman directly went to Marie-Jo to complain that I refused to help her 'because I didn't know her.' She was sobbing. Fortunately, Marie-Jo backed up my decision and helped reassure this woman that I had nonetheless found an option for her to get help on her situation. But still, I can't get over how that woman reacted yesterday." For a while, we discussed what happened, and Verthançia tried to make sense of her strong feelings about the situation. Did she feel manipulated? Did the woman strike a sensitive chord and invoke Verthançia's recurring feelings of powerlessness and guilt? "Probably she did," Verthançia acknowledged, "but I didn't feel like, not knowing this woman at all, I could just write a letter! I feel like it's also an ethical issue! Regardless, writing a letter wouldn't have changed the outcome." What Verthançia struggled with was an internal debate about whether her actions were right or wrong.

After listening, I acknowledged how difficult it must be for Verthançia to constantly encounter requests she cannot honor and how often this must happen within social work in general. Verthançia replied, "You only do this job for about ten years, and then you ask for a promotion to have an administrative position and no longer have to deal directly with service users." She also told me how much the job had changed over the past few decades: "Social workers used to have some power and leverage to change situations, to manipulate the system, but that's far from the case today."

This echoed what Marie-Jo, who started out as a social worker in the 1970s, told me one day: "That was the golden age of social work. We would write letters for service users, and that would unlock most situations."

Given tightening immigration laws and ever-decreasing resources to attend to migrants' needs, the jobs of social workers like Verthançia can seem futile today: "I fill out AME applications, I fill out CMU applications, but to me this is not doing anything. I feel like I can't do anything. People often tell me 'how lucky! What an interesting job you have!' But I tell them no, because there's nothing I can do. They don't realize what I go home with every day." Her words reminded me of research conducted by Paul Brodwin (2013) with frontline providers in United States community psychiatry. Brodwin notes that professionals become vulnerable and start grappling with a sense of futility when the ethos of their work no longer suffices, when it is no longer convincing, and when they can no longer carry out their mission or stay true to their personal ethics. They have "a sense of ineffectiveness or the felt incapacity to produce the desired result. They are forced to acknowledge the uselessness of their efforts for the task at hand, and the feeling spreads and creates doubt about the legitimacy and baseline worth of all their encounters with clients" (2013, 69).

Verthançia and I regularly work together because the social needs of migrant patients are inextricably enmeshed with the psychological ones. One day we spoke with Mrs. Adeyemi, an asylum seeker I had been seeing for therapy for almost two years. In 2015, Mrs. Adeyemi fled Nigeria because of persecutions linked to her husband's political engagement. Along with two of the couple's sons, aged fourteen and twenty, her husband had been arrested and held prisoner by the opposition party. Mrs. Adeyemi had not heard from them since, nor did she know whether they were still alive. Relatives encouraged her to flee with her youngest son, who was nine. After they applied for asylum, they accessed CADA housing. Mrs. Adeyemi's son was registered at a school, where he quickly adapted and learned French. Meanwhile, Mrs. Adeyemi showed signs of psychological distress. This motivated her social worker to refer her to Centre Minkowska.

Upon admission to the center by Dr. Bennegadi, she was diagnosed with PTSD and prescribed treatment (two antidepressants and one hypnotic). She complained of constant headaches, ruminations, sleep disorders, and chest pains. Despite her anxiety, she managed to socialize with other people at the CADA and at the local Red Cross, where she took French classes and volunteered for food distribution. Her case had been audited at OFPRA, and she was waiting for an answer. It took months for her to adjust to the treatment and observe any improvement in her health. Finally, though, she could sleep again, and her anxieties diminished. Two months later, she received a rejection letter by OFPRA. In a panic, she rushed to get a lawyer in the private sector, who required €900 (more than $1,000) to file an appeal to the CNDA. The news crushed her. She again stopped sleeping and quit her volunteer activities. It took two months for her to get an appointment at CNDA. This time, she had a Yoruba translator and felt as though she could better express her story. She said that even the president of the hearing panel noted that her narrative was clearer than initially reported by OFPRA officers. She left the court feeling "relieved" and was told she would have a response within three months. This occurred at the end of the school year, and she simultaneously received the news that her son could go to fifth grade. He was doing well at school and had received unanimous support from his teachers.

When I saw Mrs. Adeyemi at the end of the summer, she had again received a rejection letter from CNDA. Her adviser at the CADA told her that she needed to prepare for her exit. She sobbed incessantly and bent her head over her folded arms on my desk. I gave her time to gain her composure. She looked up, and her red eyes were empty with despair. I explained that increasingly, fewer refugee statuses were being awarded in France, and she would now have to pull together her remaining strength and find alternative solutions. Currently, out of the ever-increasing number of individuals rejected for asylum, only 1 percent leave the country (d'Albis and Boubtane 2018). According to a recent study, 51 percent of individuals who applied for asylum in France in 2000 had obtained a legal status for family reasons by 2016, and 32 percent were awarded a refugee status or granted subsidiary protection (d'Albis and Boubtane 2018). Legal admissions for asylum are minimal, and eventually, asylum seekers switch tactics and apply for legal status based on work- or family-related motives. This latter road to legal residency is much longer and more precarious for individuals and their families, though. They spend years living in a state of uncertainty about finding adequate housing, food, and clothing supplies and in constant fear of being arrested, detained, and deported.

I asked Mrs. Adeyemi to focus on concrete issues: preparation for her son's third year in a French school and for her emergency housing request. We brainstormed about small jobs she could find to earn some income. However, her health continued to decline, and she again had suicidal thoughts. I had Dr. Bennegadi intervene to adjust her treatment. Together, we wrote letters to local associations we knew and asked for legal and housing assistance for Mrs. Adeyemi. The goals were to keep Mrs. Adeyemi focused on concrete objectives and to avoid ruminating about being deported or living on the street with her son. I suggested she schedule an appointment with Verthançia to take stock of her social situation.

When she met with us two weeks later, she brought her son. She carried a huge plastic bag over her shoulder, and her son dragged a rolling suitcase. We learned that she had tried to commit suicide by swallowing a bottle of bleach, and she had been hospitalized and given new medication. She had also been removed from the CADA. We contacted the social worker of the district Mrs. Adeyemi lived in, who had taken over her case, but she told us there was no available space in emergency housing at that time. During the previous two nights, Mrs. Adeyemi had slept in a hospital's emergency waiting room, and her son had slept on her lap.

Verthançia let Mrs. Adeyemi know that she would have no better chance at finding housing for her, but she would try to get in touch with the social worker at her son's school to see whether they could support and prioritize Mrs. Adeyemi's housing request. After the appointment, I accompanied Mrs. Adeyemi to the waiting room. Her son waited on a chair for her, and I was overcome by sadness and a feeling of powerlessness as I held the door for them. They left the center with their "life and house" in their luggage. My throat tightened as I walked back to Verthançia's office to debrief. I found her slumped over her desk, holding her head between her hands, and she said, "This is when I hate my job. And the thing is, I feel this happens all the time. I keep telling people I have no solutions for them. At some point, it gets unbearable."

In this book, I have analyzed the ethical deliberations of Centre Minkowska staff members in MEDIACOR meetings, and I have shown that MEDIACOR offers a safe and constructive space for them to make sense of structural conundrums and assess both professional responsibility and the relevance of the referrals they receive. Obviously, staff members also face situations of suffering and injustice, created through structural inequality, in their one-on-one encounters with referred migrants. Staff members struggle to varying degrees to understand and address the complex cases they encounter, despite the deliberative outlets they have through MEDIACOR and their training in cultural competence. For example, it appears easier for Dr. Carlin to make sense of her professional world when she actively ruminates on the intersections between her personal ethics, the larger structural forces that challenge them, and her career. Her actions in the workplace are underscored by an activist drive to promote what she considers a more humane society through acts of caregiving. I argue that these acts include therapeutic forms of social support. For Verthançia, however, the reality of the clinic is more challenging—both professionally and personally. Through her experience, we glimpse what referring state agents may feel when they are confronted with patient situations that seem to fall outside their capacities for support, and how this leads to experiences of pain and impotence in the face of human despair. This is also illustrated through the case of the social worker from southern France, who desperately attempted to mobilize health professionals to help one of her critically distressed residents.

These examples demonstrate some of the challenges social workers face in general, even though they may occupy a wide array of institutional positions. In his analysis of social work as a profession, French sociologist Jean-François Gaspar (2012) identifies three ideal types of social workers: clinical, militant, and normative. Clinical social workers construe their mission as providing a response to both material and affective needs and rely on a psychosocial approach in which empathy is critical to engagement with clients. Militant social workers are particularly sensitive to the political stakes of their work and often mobilize external actors around political issues that affect clients. Finally, normative social workers are attentive to procedure, respect the legal status quo, and are generally less emotionally engaged with clients than the other two. Often, Gaspar (2012) notes, social workers straddle or are torn between these types.

I have certainly observed this tension in Verthançia's behavior and her constant struggles with feelings of futility. I have also witnessed the ways in which her role as a social worker morphs depending on her clients' situations. Some staff members at the center accuse her of aligning with Gaspar's normative understanding of a social worker and note that she seems distant with patients and colleagues alike. However, in this chapter, I have tried to present a more nuanced understanding of the experiences of staff members like Verthançia. Given her frustrations and institutional constraints, it becomes easier to understand how a more distanced position may strategically enable her to "hold on" (Gaspar 2012) in situations in which other resources—such as personal ethics, MEDIACOR team support, and administrative solutions—fall short.

*   *   *

While France has never been an ideal place of refuge and support, as it is sometimes depicted in the popular media, the past forty decades of economic recession and a weakening welfare state have negatively affected the country's structural ability to "welcome" migrants. National immigration policies oscillate between compassion and repression and are constructed around stereotyped images of migrants that fall along a dichotomy: victims who deserve care and hospitality or profiteers who threaten the country's economy. In the contemporary era, "border women/men" (Agier 2013) are placed in positions where they must find ways to survive through increasingly precarious—at times dehumanizing—social conditions. Meanwhile, state agents working in institutions dedicated to migrant care (free medical clinics, emergency housing, housing centers for asylum seekers, welfare services) are placed in positions where they must manage forms of human suffering, induced by structural conditions, in contexts characterized by increasingly limited resources, high staff turnover, and uncertainty—all of which produce ethical dilemmas and anxiety.

It is in this context that Centre Minkowska becomes a last resort, a borderland institution that offers care to those excluded from the mainstream health sector. While this humanitarian role echoes the ethos of the center's founders, it sets up a working context in which staff members are confronted daily with ethical dilemmas and frustrations. To avoid having staff members at the center become instruments of the exclusionary system they seek to subvert, the structural conditions that underpin the distressing situations of referred patients—and the very logics that underscore their referrals—must be addressed and incorporated as a major element of the cultural competence framework. In this chapter, I have shown how MEDIACOR offers a space of ethical deliberations where affective logics of work may be integrated and where, thanks to the practice of decentering, interstices of caregiving and the contestation of stigmatizing referrals may be identified.

7 · BEYOND ANXIETIES: PRAXIS

In their recent publication, *A Passion for Society*, Wilkinson and Klein-man commented that "to make possible a form of sympathetic recognition of human social situations and have this balanced alongside a rational analysis of the structural conditions that govern peoples' lives is a precarious balancing act" (2016, 155). This directly echoes what I have experienced while writing this ethnography. My goal was not to praise Centre Minkowska and its activities but to use examples from the center to advance our understanding of what factors constrain social and health-care support for migrants in a particular context. My second objective was to identify avenues for potential reform and transformation. What responsibilities do transcultural clinicians have in broader efforts to confront and to change the unjust systems of power in which they are embedded? What possibilities exist for these clinicians to make moral-agency claims that are premised on recognizing the structural constraints that animate their own professional practices? While I admit that the potential for reform and transformation is limited, at least short term, I have identified certain practices (consciousness-raising, mediating, resisting) that build on the recognition of broader structural constraints and ethical responsibility. In this chapter, I sketch the contours of a praxis that leads to more hospitable and inclusive forms of caregiving within unfair systems. Although my discussion is based on the French context, it is also relevant for other countries that face similar structural constraints and moral economies.

ANTHROPOLOGICAL THEORY AND REAL-WORLD COMPLEXITY

With this ethnography, which is based on ten years of applied work, I wished to capture real-world complexity and therefore to challenge—or to nuance—the anthropological theories I learned as a medical anthropologist. Two decades ago, when Merrill Singer and Hans Baer (1995) defined the critical medical anthropology approach, they raised an important question: Could clinical anthropology be critical? They noted that "most clinical anthropologists find themselves in the dilemma of being expected by the biomedical profession and medical institutions to serve as cultural interpreters rather than critics of existing healthcare arrangements and the large political-economic structures within which they are embedded" (Singer and Baer 1995, 352). In my own experience, I have collaborated with clinicians who worked precisely from the premise that larger structural determinants of care need to be considered in order to organize caregiving practices that can resist, if not reform, them.

My role at Centre Minkowska is not limited to that of a cultural interpreter, nor is it ambiguous. Rather, I am asked to apply the critical approach with which I entered the institution. I am also expected to highlight and to document certain aspects of care that I encounter on a daily basis: the social origins of illness, the medicalization of social problems, and the inequalities that surround health-care availability. I use my critical framework to enrich the institution's reflexive approach. At this point, the impact of my position is limited to training and research within Minkowska rather than to caregiving practices directly. In that sense, my actions in the clinic, and the clinical medical anthropology model that informs Minkowska's caregiving practices, certainly fall short of Nancy Scheper-Hughes's (1990) call for a critically applied medical anthropology that entails revolutionary changes. But does that mean the clinical-anthropology-inspired mission at Centre Minkowska is limited to questioning how to care for patients who need immediate medical assistance or to "patching" problems (Waitzkin 1983)—a practice that tends to misrecognize sociocultural inequalities?

I find the critical medical and critical moral anthropology frameworks limiting in some ways: both frameworks leave researchers within a narrowly political frame and suggest—rightfully—that the very initiatives of humanitarian, compassionate action and practice that we study are constrained by regulatory policing frameworks that are bound to reproduce existing social inequalities (Fassin 2012; Ticktin 2011). I cannot say that I have never wrestled with the idea that the work done at Centre Minkowska or at other similar "borderland" institutions is a two-pronged system in which some people are deemed more deserving of care than others. As I have shown in this ethnography, the double binds that Minkowska professionals recurrently face are emblematic of this very idea. Because this possibility is acknowledged rather than disavowed at the center, though, I suggest that interstices may be identified where structural inequalities—and the differential practices they produce—may be contested. Some people may argue that the mere act of recognition or of contestation depoliticizes the clinical encounter and that my position—or that of my colleagues—equates to promoting the status quo. However, I show how we, as field professionals, are involved in moral economies that transcend the work we do, and this need not limit our potential to explore alternative clinical paradigms.

LESSONS FOR IMPROVING CAREGIVING PRACTICES

In this ethnography, I do not limit myself to exploring the practice of cultural competence—as it is applied at Centre Minkowska—in search of lessons for critical theory only. I also discuss lessons for social justice and for improved caregiving practices. I focus on migrants, but the broader themes I tackle relate to other people, as well; in some ways, migrants act as a magnifying glass for all people who find themselves in situations of extreme vulnerability. In fact, current caregiving market models, as they are applied in the United States or in the United Kingdom, place us all at risk for vulnerability and precarity when we experience ill health. Notably, these market models increasingly erode the French tradition of social medicine.

I discuss here three main lessons: First, social inequalities are inextricably related to health issues. Second, biomedicine (psychiatry in particular) can address the overlap between social inequality and health in only limited ways when it is implemented alone. Third, social inequalities that are based on stigmatizing representations and on unequal access to resources negatively affect both patients and providers. From these lessons, it becomes clear that health-care policies need to facilitate and to implement dialogues between social and health services. Policies also need to be created that normalize professional training in both social and health services through methods informed by a larger implementation framework that transcends disciplinary boundaries.

In this respect, my ethnography relates to global (mental) health issues; I establish how mental illness stems from living within social inequality and how, as a consequence, treatment approaches need to address discriminatory barriers to care and the institutional maltreatment of both patients and their caretakers (Kohrt and Mendenhall 2015). Mental health issues have gained visibility in the past decade partly because of WHO's (2001, 2010) increasing attention to the issue, but this visibility has not yet led to firm implementation paths that challenge inequalities in access to mental health care. In *Cultural Anxieties*, I show how legislative attention to migrants' traumas often fails to be translated into practice in France—and in Europe more generally—because it does not attend to structural constraints or to professional training.

Addressing Structural Constraints

For years, medical anthropologists have identified the roots of structural violence and their relationships to health inequalities (Farmer 2004). Some anthropologists, such as Paul Farmer, have worked in the field as clinicians and have proposed to incorporate structural interventions into their medical and public health practices (Farmer et al. 2006). So far, the results from these efforts seem limited to local initiatives, such as Farmer's Partners in Health program. Within French anthropology, critiques of health policies abound (Fassin and Dozon 2001; Fassin and Rechtman 2009), but they have resulted in few proposed public health alternatives that translate field observations into innovative programs. I suggest that this is partly due to the wider gap that exists in France between academia and applied work.

Until recently, public health policy related to immigration and to caregiving practices for migrants has seldom acknowledged or considered social determinants such as housing and living conditions, access to welfare services, and administrative hardships. Medical anthropologists have therefore encouraged public health practitioners and policy makers to examine immigration "as both socially determined and a social determinant of health" (Castañeda et al. 2015, 376). Rather than depicting migrants as an *at-risk* population, which places responsibility on individuals, researchers argue that it is preferable to identify migrants as "structurally vulnerable" (Quesada, Hart, and Bourgois 2011).

Within the French public health system, understandings of the social determinants of disease and of suffering have resulted in the development of specific clinical approaches and dedicated health-care services since the 1990s. The emergence of a *new poverty* (Paugam 1991) and its resultant psychological suffering, which is linked to the erosion of the social protection system and to successive unemployment crises over the past forty years, mobilized psychiatrists around the notion of *psycho-social suffering* (Furtos 2008). This, in turn, led to the creation of listening units (*lieux d'écoute*) at the intersection of mental health and social work, which were tasked with creating new approaches to mental health that did not necessarily resort to mental health professionals but relied instead on social workers or special educators. In his analysis of this phenomenon, Didier Fassin (2006) noted that many psychiatrists were engaged in theorizing this new form of expertise at a policy level, but very few of them were involved in its application in practice. As for psychologists, they increasingly competed with social workers to perform missions for which they were not trained, such as organizing educational activities or undertaking administrative tasks (Fassin 2006).

Meanwhile, the national management of welfare services has radically transformed over recent decades. Management transitioned from local NGOs—which mobilized moral values related to volunteer work, Catholicism, and scouting—to decentralized, privately run institutions, which mobilized market-oriented logics and business ethics of efficiency and profit (Bouquet 2006). In addition, in response to multiple forms of prior social exclusion, welfare services became hyperspecialized in form (disability, exclusion, socialization, compensation, prevention, family support), targets (childhood, families, the elderly), and means (from social engineering to psychological support) (Bouquet 2006, 127). This fragmentation of welfare services has detrimentally affected the quality of social work and of caregiving practices in France.

A PSYCHOPATHOLOGIZATION OF SOCIAL SUFFERING?

Besides the reification of cultural identities in interpretations of "migrant suffering," a central issue I have tackled in this book is the psychopathologization of social suffering. Just as it has emerged in this ethnography, mental health actors have observed the psychopathologization of social suffering in their own work. From this perspective, the psychosocial intervention, as articulated in transcultural clinics, enables a form of politicization: it acknowledges that problems are not solely related to individuals' personality traits but to the circumstances within which individuals live. In the research she conducted on clinical interactions at Centre Minkowska, clinical psychologist and anthropologist Daria Rostirolla (2017) reminds us that it is illusory to separate considerations of individuals and of society and that, in the therapeutic context, a clinical anthropology approach that is sensitive to contemporary forms of suffering necessarily apprehends subjects within their relational "configurations" (2017, 282–283). Expressions of suffering that relate to disruptions in social relations and to social inequalities, Rostirolla argues, allow clinicians to question clinical interventions and to think of individuals' demands within a web of larger social determinants.

Transcultural clinics and the anthropological model that underpins them allow professionals to move beyond social categories and to approach migrants as subjects; professionals can transcend the administrative limits that are imposed on them and that are necessary for the state institutions that support them to function (e.g., categories such as "asylum seeker," "unaccompanied minor," "refugee," and "Dublined"). This includes the most recent social constructions of vulnerability, which risk generating another scale of deservingness as they are reclaimed by the policies on asylum, as we saw in chapter 6. Typically, when health practitioners in France use the term "vulnerabilities," they refer to situations and not to groups—that is, an individual may seem vulnerable if the situations the individual experienced had traumatic or pathological repercussions. But the action of tying the notion of vulnerability to a category of people produces a hierarchy of rights that may be problematic for clinicians. In this respect, the transcultural clinic offers a protected space where individuals—both professionals and patients—may free themselves from assigned, exclusionary social spaces. This certainly echoes Eugène Minkowski's approach to psychotherapy—not for its politics but for its attempt to elude the psychological categories that limit understandings of individuals' experiences.

SYSTEMIC INTERVENTION

I am well aware that in the United States, scholars have lodged critiques against the cultural competence model. These critiques position the model as limiting its focus to the clinical encounter—and therefore overlooking how broader social, economic, and political conditions produce health inequalities—and as limiting its corrective actions outside the clinic walls (Metzl and Hansen 2014, 2018). In addition, some scholars speak of cultural humility rather than cultural competence and emphasize how important it is for professionals to practice self-awareness and reflection. Several scholars have made suggestions for promoting corrective actions, such as acting on curricula (Hansen, Braslow, and Rohrbaugh 2018) and promoting advocacy (Kirmayer, Kronick, and Rousseau 2018). Readers will attest that the aforementioned critiques are incorporated into Centre Minkowska's cultural competence model and that our person-centered approach does not limit our focus to the clinical encounter; rather, our approach aims to address stigma, which is prevalent in transcultural interactions. It may be debated whether we should change our terminology; semantics *do* in fact matter. Perhaps what matters most, at this point, is clarifying methodological actions and identifying avenues through which cultural competence may lead to systemic intervention.

Education and Professional Training Are Key

In medical schools in France, there are fewer opportunities to integrate social theory and clinical practice than there are in U.S. programs, such as Harvard Medical School's Global Health and Social Medicine program or the psychiatry residency programs at New York University, the University of California–Los Angeles, and Yale University (Hansen, Braslow, and Rohrbaugh 2018, 117). In France, integrative efforts are usually practiced by professionals, and they tend to access information about such integration through the few existing continuing education programs on the topic—such as the one we offer in partnership with Université Paris Descartes. For psychology and psychiatry interns who become interested in transcultural psychiatry, MEDIACOR offers a unique setting in which clinical trainees may observe the multidimensional logics of health-care interactions and may learn to analyze situations from a global health perspective. Introducing theses trainees to the clinical medical anthropology model also enables them to apprehend illness in the context of structural factors beyond the clinical encounter.

During our latest training for CADA professionals on how to identify and cope with residents' psychotraumas, Verthançia and I organized a joint program in which we integrated the local realities and constraints of our trainees in order to identify local stakeholders, institutional resources, and concrete strategies for organizing community intervention. This led us to travel to the northern half of France. Because France decentralized CADAs—until recently, they were grouped in the Paris area—professionals struggle to find local resources for organizing health support (especially for psychiatric follow-up, as illustrated in chapter 6). In this context, professional training may offer practical tools for improving access to services. Such training may also offer tools to help institution staff members—who are sometimes unfamiliar with how to welcome vulnerable populations, such as asylum seekers—identify resources for building inclusive health and social practices.

Crossing Boundaries and Promoting Pluridisciplinarity

From my experience at Centre Minkowska, I have observed that one way for people to more effectively address structural constraints is to foster an ability to cross boundaries and to work in an interdisciplinary manner. I have argued that being situated at the borderland resulted in both positive and negative impacts. On the negative end, working at the interstices of health care often resulted in Centre Minkowska acting as a stopgap. On the positive end, working from that position placed the center at the intersection of discourses and practices that fostered interdisciplinarity and boundary crossing.

To some extent, these dynamics are inherent to the transcultural clinic space. In her ethnography of the Italian ethnopsychiatry clinic Centre Fanon, anthropologist Cristiana Giordano analyzed how professionals are "being pushed to cross thresholds when working with foreigners (disciplinary, vocational and professional), entailing a critique of boundaries between different domains of knowledge and practice" (2014, 109). Ultimately, the transcultural clinic provoked a new approach to professionals' work and led them to question the state's project of integration and multiculturalism (Giordano 2014, 109). To this I would add that crossing professional and disciplinary boundaries also fosters professionals' ability to see "the big picture," and it opens their minds to the structural dimensions of health.

At a conference I attended a few years ago, organized by Marie Rose Moro's transcultural clinic,[1] we reflected on the contribution of the transcultural approach to the treatment of chronic diseases and to the ways in which therapeutic education programs are construed. We concluded that the obstacles encountered in the context of transcultural care and the solutions found to solve them significantly contributed to re-centering patients as the focus of care programs, and to promoting interdisciplinarity. Solutions relied on the intervention of cultural mediators and the application of a structural approach to health. Transcultural care practice considers a patient's personal, social, and professional environments; this highlights the limits of the biomedical model. Transcultural care practice values an individual's experiential knowledge and positions it as expertise. These (and other) major strides in care were partly derived from transcultural care contributions in the domains of HIV/AIDS, diabetes, cancer, and psychological/psychiatric disorders. At a recent conference organized by the association of PASS clinics—another "borderland" institution[2]—participants asked similar questions and drew similar conclusions: How do these specific caregiving units welcome those who are socially excluded and who have no health-care coverage? How do they become the most hospitable units at hospitals? Staff members at PASS clinics face issues similar to those faced by transcultural clinicians. An important one is the question of patient triage. Both types of professionals are constrained by hospital budget allocations; they engage their colleagues across services through pluridisciplinary collaborations, and they create bridges within the hospitals in which they work and with social and medical actors outside hospital walls.

As I discussed in chapter 2, interdisciplinarity rests at the heart of Centre Minkowska's continuing education program; both our students (from all sectors of medicine, social work, education, and justice) and our teachers (from anthropology, medicine, social work, education, and justice) come from diverse fields. This diversity fosters conversation among all areas of social life and leads professionals to develop an acute understanding of the constraints their patients and colleagues face when they address health issues.

Research and Advocacy

By linking clinical activities to research, teaching, and professional training, Centre Minkowska is in a unique position to promote advocacy—that is, to work with institutions to change clinical practices and ultimately to influence health policy (Kirmayer, Kronick, and Rousseau 2018, 119). Our daily interactions with referring professionals across health and social sectors provide opportunities to identify systemic failures and to imagine strategies to take corrective actions.

The issue of interpreters, for example, is one that has slowly emerged as a public health concern, primarily because transcultural institutions like Centre Minkowska have contributed to making the issue visible to health authorities. In chapter 3, I explored how language obstacles and state institutions' unwillingness or inability to work with professional interpreters account for a majority of migrants' health inequalities and for most instances of unequal access to health care and social services. The referrals screened during MEDIACOR allowed us to identify, disturbingly, that most district CMPs turned down referrals for non-francophone patients and systematically referred them to Centre Minkowska. In chapter 5, I introduced the action-research we implemented from this clinical observation. This research was small in scale, but it had a tremendous impact: two-thirds of the institutions with whom we worked doubled their budgets for interpreters and now often ask how they ever worked without this critical type of facilitator. To further advocate for this issue, we organized a conference at the Ministry of Health and invited participating CMP professionals and interpreters to share their experiences about how this change had improved their caregiving practices. In the aftermath of this project, we were also contacted by the Regional Health Agency and asked to help them identify resources that would facilitate access to professional interpreters in health. This illustrates how even local actions can lead to change in policy and practice.

MEDIACOR interventions are another example of advocacy. Since MEDIACOR was identified as a resource for an increasing number of professionals outside the center, the unit has helped other institutions solve complex situations without resorting to patient referrals. This means that by integrating and communicating with community actors, the deliberative setting at Centre

Minkowska harbors great potential for systemic action and change, and it seems to me that the time is ripe to think about ways to promote this experience on a larger scale. For example, rather than limiting its scope to internal staff meetings on patient triage, MEDIACOR could open its doors to outside professionals and provide an external deliberation platform to enable earlier interventions in caregiving practices for migrant populations. Such a change has the potential to prevent the now common "vagrant" therapeutic itineraries that tend to worsen vulnerable patients' health and complicate social and health service provision.

HOSPITABLE PRACTICES AND THE AFFECTIVE LOGICS OF CAREGIVING

In this book, I argue that cultural competence as enacted at Centre Minkowska—through the practice of deliberating and decentering—provides the essential fuel needed to work toward social justice and to implement hospitable practices. Hospitable practices are those that create humane and empathetic interstices of action and caregiving, that nourish the possibility of finding meaning in one's work, and that foster the necessary energy to take action. Here I argue that the transcultural clinic—and other borderland institutions like it—serves as a laboratory where a politics of hospitality can be tested. I do not think of hospitality as yet another illusory and politically ineffective normative horizon amid the compassion moral economy. Rather, I think of it as a concept to be directly applied to practice (Chambon 2017, Le Blanc and Brugère 2017).

In many ways, my vision of hospitable practice relates to the ethics of hospitality as they were articulated by philosophers Emmanuel Levinas ([1961] 1991) or Jacques Derrida and Anne Dufourmantelle (1997), but it seeks to adapt these ethics' unconditional vision to the reality of institutional constraints. In my practical take on these ethics, through the world of health and social-work professionals, I think of hospitality as relying first and foremost on empathy and on an ability to cross boundaries, or to tolerate having one's boundaries crossed. As is visible through this ethnography, in the face of the multiple anxieties experienced by professionals working with vulnerable populations, this type of empathy is tested daily. Within the institutions of the referring actors and state agents I mentioned throughout this book, certain constraints—managerial policies, work fragmentation, and budget restrictions—often cause professionals to experience burnout and to lose their sense of the value of their work. In this context, it is understandably difficult to find the necessary energy to face and to sort out complex situations. It also makes sense, then, that expressions of difference—however they are expressed—directly challenge hospitality and potentially transform it into hostility. In chapter 6, we saw how these difficulties occur even in the hospitable and flexible space of the transcultural clinic. Based on my experience and on the analysis I have offered throughout this book, I argue that there are two essential ingredients for promoting hospitable practices: fostering professionals' moral agency and implementing techniques to deconstruct social categories.

Professionals' Moral Agency

Recent ethnographies have analyzed "moral agency" as a person's ability to live a "good life," which entails making intimate connections with others and being recognized as a "good" person by those who occupy the same local moral world (e.g., Garcia 2010; Myers 2015). Caregiving itself is a moral experience: as Arthur Kleinman notes, "What is at stake is doing good for oneself and for others" (2012, 1551). In *Cultural Anxieties*, I define the moral agency of an individual as the person's ability to reconcile his or her personal and professional ethics of care and responsibility with everyday practices. As I illustrated in chapter 6, this moral agency is constrained by a person's professional status, gender, and age, and it can be limited when a rupture exists between the person's ideals and everyday practice. I argue that to be able to provide humane caregiving, professionals need to find a sense of moral agency.

Admittedly, fostering moral agency among professionals may be the trickiest piece of this praxis puzzle to achieve—the main reason being that moral agency is multifactorial and is inextricably linked to improving the unfair system in which professionals are embedded and which inspires feelings of futility when working with vulnerable populations like migrants, more than it promotes moral agency (Coutant and Eideliman 2013; for examples in American psychiatric contexts, see Brodwin 2013; DelVecchio Good et al. 2001). Benefiting from group and individual supervision and participating in strategies for corrective action are what allow professionals to maintain a sense of purpose in their work. As this ethnography demonstrates, this may be particularly challenging for professionals working in state institutions, where many experience a sense of isolation and end up questioning the effectiveness or the very meaning of their actions. The situation of the referring social worker for Hamza in chapter 6 provides one edifying illustration. At this point, we cannot expect the state to implement hospitable practices (Le Blanc and Brugère 2017). However, as transcultural professionals who benefit from the flexibility of our borderland position, we may think of local and small-scale inclusive projects that may build positive collective experience from the ground up. Based on the MEDIACOR model, this could take the shape of a collective space or deliberative unit where isolated state professionals could gather or find resources to overcome the obstacles they meet in everyday practice. Such a collective platform could lead to identifying and coordinating individual strategies for corrective action, which in turn could progressively transform institutional practices.

Deconstructing Social Categories

With respect to migrants, I suggest that the transcultural paradigm, with its anthropological premise, may achieve caregiving through its reflexive approach; the paradigm teaches people how to deconstruct identity categories and, in this way, to recognize the political dimension of caregiving.

The transcultural approach is a good antidote for France's schizophrenic posture toward its multicultural identity and for societies that fear the invasion of "migrant others." The prefix "trans-" popularly denotes notions of "across" or "through"—the idea that there is not a perfectly homogeneous inside or outside—an "us" versus a "them." From an anthropological perspective, as Michel Agier (2013) has shown in his work on the cosmopolitan condition, borders have been instrumental to humans as "elementary structures" that aid people in their attempts to construe social identities and to relate to others. Some individuals benefit from occupying liminal, border states in order to negotiate their own identities. In the end, "we have always been border-beings" (*des êtres de frontière*) (Mbembe 2016, 46; my translation). The transcultural clinic offers a safe space within which a person may dismantle "racist fears" (Mbembe 2016, 113) inherited from the colonial past and identify related projections that place others at a safe distance or that turn others into scapegoats.

By deconstructing social categories, the transcultural clinic constitutes a space in which individuals are acknowledged in their humanity, the frontiers of identity are contested, and therapists in training and referring state agents who attend MEDIACOR sessions are able to learn to decenter and to think critically about social complexity and structural constraints. This feels difficult, as it entails accepting one's own vulnerability in the face of what may feel like unacceptable, strange, and unsolvable problems. But it is this very act of recognition—of acknowledging cultural difference, structural constraints, and one's vulnerability—that may enable hospitality.

CONCLUSION

The anxieties surrounding the efforts of referring social actors to manage "migrant suffering"—whether they relate to the political characterization of migrants themselves, to the scarcity conditions social actors face at work, to social actors' capacities to relate to migrants, or to all of these combined—are expressed in the transcultural clinic at Centre Minkowska. In turn, these anxieties raise questions about transcultural clinicians' own ethics and bring up issues of responsibility and of hospitality in health care—and in society more broadly. In fact, beyond relating to migrants, such anxieties raise questions about how we have come to relate to our own humanity and vulnerability.

The roots of this social situation are so deep and spread so far that it inspires a feeling of vertigo. There is an increasing number of social inequalities that everyone seems able to denounce—those that fuel violence, poverty, and migration all over the world. Beyond those, however, are other equally pervasive inequalities that have deeply affected migrants in the French context. In particular, I draw attention to the consequences of structural adjustment programs, which were layered over decades of human, environmental, and economic spoilage during colonization. Today, migration itself fuels a thriving transnational economy that spans from smugglers to security companies. However, we are in a self-destructive spiral: our economic system consumes us and turns us into slaves not only of certain types of social organization—work-pace acceleration, extreme consumerism, and weakening solidarities—but of a particular brand of subverted ethics. Our economic system directly influences our moral stances, including those related to whom we characterize as worth our care and compassion and whose lives we position as valuable. In this ethnography, I have illustrated how the lives of some contemporary migrants epitomize the outcomes of this self-destructive system.

Through questioning its violent and complex colonial origins, Centre Minkowska was gradually able to reconsider migrants as social figures—both as *objects* of alterity, individuals whose basic rights are negated, and as *subjects*, people who question their own alterity. In the genealogy offered in this book, I have identified historical transitions between different modes of subordinating (and governing) migrants through regimes of cultural representation: from labor migrants to economic migrants, from refugees to asylum seekers, and from undocumented migrants to precarious migrants. These transitions have provided opportunities to critically reflect on clinical modalities and on the ways in which health professionals relate to people designated "other." The development of the clinical medical anthropology model and the related cultural competence approach at Centre Minkowska attests to this reflexive process.

The center's approach, I argue, contributes to practical routes for strengthening migrant care in three major ways: First, it offers training to help professionals broaden their expert gazes in order to recognize the external, systemic causes behind failures in institutional care or support and to help them understand the basics of working in a transcultural context—such as the importance of interpreters. Second, it provides a safe environment in which people may confront many different explanatory models of health and of suffering and in which they may practice reflexivity. In particular, this environment is promoted by MEDIACOR meetings through the practice of deliberation, which fosters pluridisciplinarity in exchanges and positions cultural competence as a sense-making framework rather than a normative practice. This deliberative space becomes especially important when transcultural professionals' ideals are confronted with the violence of structural inequalities and the challenges of addressing the systemic needs of their patients. Finally, through action-research projects and MEDIACOR community outreach, the center promotes advocacy, which aims to improve care by influencing policy and increasing resources for migrants.

The clinical medical anthropology model developed at Centre Minkowska reminds us that two things in particular *matter*: interpreting situations from a global perspective and focusing on relationships of caregiving. The political project, then, is not to naively promote a common humanity (as normative ethics often does) but to recognize differences in order to allow them to coexist. The work of mediating and deliberating in the transcultural clinic necessitates reinvesting in what I call the affective logics of caregiving: a work of posture that enables a person to manage uncertainty and to accept a position of "not-knowing" when he or she faces difference or structural complexity. This, in turn, allows professionals to move beyond anxieties and to understand that when caring for "others," we also care for ourselves.

ACKNOWLEDGMENTS

First and foremost, I am deeply grateful to my colleagues at Centre Minkowska. My gratitude goes to Rachid Bennegadi, Marie-Jo Bourdin, and Christophe Paris for taking a chance on hiring an anthropologist and for defending the relevance of my presence inside the clinic. This book builds on the engaged and generous work of my colleagues at the center: Maria Vittoria Carlin, Smaïl Cheref, Audrey Gittinger, Christine Pinto Lenoir, Verthançia Mavanga, Daria Rostirolla, and Laetitia Virgal. Through this book, I want to pay tribute to all of them.

As this is only one part of the center's team, I would also like to acknowledge the contributions of the remainder of Centre Minkowska's staff: Soraya Ayouch, Nader Barzin, Jenny Voltaire, Mika Delpierre, Maurice Dores, Maja Guberina, Afrodita Hodza, Christophe Huby, Kouakou Kouassi, Can Liem Luong, Georges Meliz, Maruca Mendieta, Benan Penpe-Ozer, Doudou Sarr, and Ines De Paula Vasques.

I also want to pay tribute to the patients and the professional interpreters I have been fortunate to work with at the center. Practicing in a transcultural context with people who come from a variety of cultures and life experiences is both incredibly enriching and humbling.

This professional and intellectual venture germinated almost two decades ago, when I arrived at Southern Methodist University in Dallas to start a graduate program in anthropology. I had freshly graduated from the MAPPS program at the University of Chicago, and I was interested in transnationalism and identity transformation in the context of migration. I knew little about medical anthropology, and I did not anticipate working on migration-related health issues. As these things often do, this new orientation in my life began with an encounter. Medical anthropologist Carolyn Sargent has been a true mentor and friend, and she offered me this wonderful opportunity of doing fieldwork at home while studying abroad. Through the years, Carolyn has continued offering me professional support and advice, and I am extremely grateful to her for that as well. At SMU, I benefited from the great mentorship of Carolyn Smith-Morris and Caroline Brettell. Two other SMU scholars who have since passed away also had an influence on my training: Victoria Lockwood and Robert Van Kemper.

While in France, Carolyn introduced me to anthropology and sociology colleagues at CRESP (Centre de recherche sur la santé, le social et le politique): a research center on health, society, and politics, which was created by Didier Fassin. This opened up another opportunity for me—that of completing a joint degree at EHESS (Ecole des hautes études en sciences sociales) in Paris under Didier Fassin's supervision. It was a chance for me to benefit from the close supervision of a scholar whose work had inspired my research in France. I would like to express my gratitude to him again, through this book, for welcoming me at EHESS with his students at the IRIS research center (replacing CRESP) and for his mentorship during my doctoral studies.

After my fieldwork, I went to Washington University in Saint Louis to complete my dissertation and found a very supportive and intellectually stimulating environment. I am extremely grateful to the university's School of Social Sciences and the Department of Anthropology for funding the remainder of my graduate years. At WashU, I benefited from wonderful mentorships with scholars who became part of my jury committee: John Bowen, Rebecca Lester, and Brad Stoner. I also want to acknowledge the witty support and humor of my writing workshop friends—among them Meghan Ferrence, Katie Hejtmanek, and Anna Jacobsen, as well as of my gourmet partners, Mary Jane Acuña and Abby Stone. I also benefited from the insights of other talented scholars in the anthropology department; among them, I want to thank Stephen Scott, who influenced my analysis on language in this book, as well as Robert Sussman and Tab Rassmussen, two renowned physical anthropologists who have unfortunately passed away.

After completing my PhD and returning to France, I faced the challenge of carrying out the duties of my then part-time position at Centre Minkowska along with my postdoctoral activities. I was fortunate to be invited by Laurence Kotobi, my colleague and friend from Université de Bordeaux, to work on a project on the role of interpreters in breaking bad news in oncological care. This was an opportunity to continue exploring the relevance of professional interpreters in health institutions, and I gained tremendous insight for the pursuit of my career in the transcultural clinic. I am indebted to Laurence for her continuous professional support and friendship.

Many other collaborations followed, with wonderful scholars and clinicians from Canada, Switzerland, France, and the United States. Among them I would like to thank Zahia Kessar, Isabelle Marin, Idriss Farota-Romejko, Denis Mechali, Melissa Dominice Dao, Patricia Hudelson, Orest Weber, Yvan Leanza, Barbara Rylko-Bauer, Eric Jarvis, Margareth Zanchetta, Ismaël Maiga, Sarah Willen, Serge Bouznah, Marie Rose Moro, Gesine Sturm, Marguerite Coignet, Richard Rechtman, Mahamet Timera, and Ahmet Karamustafa. I am also indebted to the students and professionals I met along the way, as well as to the GERMES group at Université Paris Diderot, which became my academic home after I returned to France.

In 2015, I was elected president of ISM-Interprétariat, a nonprofit association providing professional translation and interpreting services to French state institutions. This position provided me with tremendous insight into the work and constraints of professional interpreters and into the logics of funding such services, which I partly address in this book. I would particularly like to express my gratitude to the director at ISM, Aziz Tabouri, for supporting my activities and this book project.

For helping me find the courage to write this book and encourage me through the process, I am thankful to my peers and teachers at the EEPA school of psychotherapy in Paris (Ecole Européenne des philosophies et psychothérapie appliquées), especially Anita Pinato and Marianne Quiles. I am equally thankful to Nicole Aknin, director of the Sigmund Freud University in Paris, for offering me an opportunity to teach there and be in regular conversation with students in psychology.

At Rutgers University Press, I thank Lenore Manderson, editor of this series, for supporting this book and for her careful editorial work and comments. I am also very grateful to Rutgers's editorial director, Kimberly Guinta, whom I first met at a AAA conference, and who took the time to listen to me and to consider relaying my project to the press. Thank you so much for your availability and flexibility during the writing process. In the last stage of this writing adventure, I also benefited from the meticulous editorial work of Jessica Ruthven. I am extremely grateful to Jessica for her level of engagement with the material. She was very influential in helping me bring out the ethnography when I was tempted to drift toward theoretical considerations. To the extent that I was successful in achieving a balance between both, I owe her.

He will likely never come across this book, but my appreciation goes to Toumani Diabate and his kora music for helping me concentrate on writing. I also want to express my most sincere gratitude to Marie-Laure Héricourt for her kind and generous guidance through the years.

Marie Labaeye Bryche, Katie Hejtmanek, Dorra Mameri-Chaambi, Rachel Wadoux, Idriss Farota-Romejko, Daria Rostirolla, and Ursula Acklin Kalil—my friends over many years—have been sources of steady encouragement. I am fortunate to have these beautiful souls in my life! Daria and Jesper, special thanks for welcoming us into your beautiful Norwegian cabin and providing me with breathtaking, inspiring mountain scenery for the very last writing stage of this book.

Last but not least, I would like to thank my parents, Michel and Marie-Claude Larchanché; my sister, Elodie Larchanché; and my brother-in-law, Jean-Raymond Odabachian, for their unwavering support and love. My daughter, Julia, is herself a source of inspiration for this book, and I know that when the time comes for her to read it, she will understand why. But ultimately, I would not have been able to complete this book without the loving partnership of my husband, Zanga-dit-Drissa Dembele. Your love, patience, understanding, and infallible availability as both a parent and a partner were the essential ingredients for this book to come to life. *Ne bi fe.*

NOTES

INTRODUCTION

1. The Kayes region is the most western region of Mali, at the border of Mauritania and Senegal. It is largely rural and poor, and it has been a historic place of immigration to France.
2. As do most of my colleagues, I alternate referring to Centre Minkowska as the Centre or as Minkowska.
3. The Centre has three domains of activity: the clinic, research and teaching, and professional training. For more details, visit the website at www.minkowska.com.

1. A GENEALOGY OF "MIGRANT SUFFERING"

1. Racist representations of North Africans have informed representations in France's contemporary public imaginary, which casts them as religiously fanatic and violent individuals. This is particularly apparent in representations of North African youth.
2. The hospital's architects incorporated some elements of North African architecture into the hospital structure. They built a monumental Moorish style entrance, evocative of North African culture. In 1935, shortly after the completion of the hospital, a project for a Muslim cemetery was initiated. Indeed, North African workers, who often migrated alone in conditions of poverty and isolation, sometimes died in France without the possibility of being offered a proper Muslim burial, or their families could not afford the repatriation of their bodies. The Seine Regional Council thus offered the hospital an adjacent four-acre piece of land, and the Muslim cemetery was inaugurated in 1937. All these initiatives were aimed at polishing the image of France as a benevolent and powerful empire (Musée de l'Assistance Publique—Hôpitaux de Paris 2005).
3. I emphasize the concepts of "emigration" and "immigration" to underline Sayad's efforts at showing how the distinction between the two is overlooked in public discourse on immigrants and their living conditions.
4. In France, the Waldeck-Rousseau law of 1901 allows citizens to form voluntary associations. Depending on the nature of their projects and activities, associations may receive funding from one to several sources at the state, regional, or local level. The 1905 law on the separation of church and state allowed religions to organize as private associations as well (see Bowen 2007). Associations recognized by the state as being of "public utility" (*associations reconnues d'utilité publique*) may benefit from greater state funding. The creation of associations has grown in popularity throughout the twentieth century in France, especially since the end of World War II. More associations were created in the last thirty years than since 1901, and it has been estimated that approximately seventy thousand associations are created each year. Today, France counts approximately one million active associations, most of which are related to cultural activities (15%), followed by health or social services (8%) and education, training, or housing services (7%) (Ministère de la Jeunesse et des Sports 2010). Since 1981, foreign residents also have the right to form associations. This has led to a proliferation of immigrant associations, which most commonly focus on sponsoring initiatives within sending communities (see Daum 1998); organizing cultural activities for immigrant communities in France; providing legal, social, and health services to legal and undocumented immigrants; and encouraging citizenship participation for "children of immigrants" (see Ricardou and Yatera 2007 on youth of sub-Saharan African origin).

5. This refers to riots in the suburbs of Lyon in 1981.

6. Stipends for the unemployed were a result of the creation of the income support allowance (RMI—Revenu Minimum d'Insertion) in 1988.

7. Fassin et al. (2004, 24) point to two reports in particular: *Exclus et exclusion* (1991) by Philippe Nasse and *Cohésion sociale et prévention de l'exclusion* by Bertrand Fragonard.

8. Devereux argued that it is impossible to dissociate the study of culture from that of the psyche, because both are concepts that, although distinct, are complementary to each other. Culture and psyche should be considered as two facets of the same reality, presupposing each other reciprocally, both functionally and methodologically. Hence the need for a complementarity between psychoanalysis and ethnology (Devereux 1980). This complementarity is only possible because Devereux made a careful distinction between a universal expression of "culture in itself" (or *metaculture*) and local expressions of culture. Like psychiatrists, Devereux adhered to the principle of a universal psyche, to which the concept of culture relates: "Indeed, regardless of the variety of cultures," he wrote, "the simple fact of having a culture is a genuinely universal experience, and man functions as a 'creator, creature, manipulator, and transmitter of culture' (Simmons 1942) everywhere and in the same way" (1980, 69). This made it possible for psychiatrists to also engage with the practice of ethnopsychiatry.

9. "Second intention" is a French public health term indicating that patients do not come for a consultation on their own initiative. Rather, their pathology is first suspected by one institution (such as those mentioned in the text), which then contacts the deemed appropriate health structure for consultation.

10. The trials against excision began in 1983, the 1989 "headscarf affair" led to a law in 2004 banning the wearing of conspicuous religious symbols, and the anti-polygamy laws were established in 1993.

11. See the famous comment Chirac made during a right-wing party meeting on the need to reframe immigration policies: "How do you want a French worker who works with his wife, earning together about 15,000 FF (about 2,300 euros), and who sees on the floor of his low-income high-rise (HLM), all piled-up, a family with a father, three or four spouses and twenty children earning 50,000 FF (almost 8,000 euros) only from social benefits, and naturally without working. . . . If you add to that the noise and the smell, well the French worker, he goes mad. And it is not racist to say this. We no longer have the means of pursuing the family reunification policy, and we need to finally tackle the essential debate in this country, as to whether it is moral and normal that foreigners should profit, to the same extent as French people, from a national solidarity to which they don't participate, as they pay no income taxes" (*L'Humanité* 1991).

12. Public intervention at a seminar on mental health and immigration, Maison des Sciences de l'Homme, St. Denis, September 1, 2008.

2. TRANSCULTURAL PRACTICE AT CENTRE MINKOWSKA

1. The systemic approach is based on systems theory, and construes patients as part of a broader system in which actors and the environment are interdependent and interrelated. In this perspective, a therapist will try to identify factors that may be related to a patient's reported symptoms: the patient's family system, friends, culture, and communication dynamics; the education system; the natural environment; and so on.

2. Following the deinstitutionalization of psychiatry in 1960, the dominant model in the organization of comprehensive psychiatric care in France has been the creation of geographically defined areas, known as sectors. Community-based (or sector-based) mental health care was born out of concerns with the continuity of care, the development of partnerships with

patients and families, and the involvement of the local community. In this system, psychiatry has become one among various mental health therapeutic options, such as psychotherapy, art therapy, and occupational therapy. Community-based mental health care has also sought the integration of mental health care into primary health care, along with the provision of social services, such as employment and housing. In French public health jargon, a community mental health institution is referred to as a *centre medico-psychologique*, or CMP (literally, "medicopsychological center"). In Paris, each arrondissement is divided into several geographic sectors, each of which has a CMP.

3. All public health institutions in France must elect a board of representatives for their medical staff. The CME is an advisory body for health-care provision and medical staff management issues.

3. CULTURAL AND LINGUISTIC DIFFERENCE AS OBSTACLES TO CARE

1. Inter-Migrant Services is an association created in 1970. It provides translation and interpreting services on the phone, on-site, and now via videoconference in over a hundred languages and dialects. IMS provides most translating and interpreting services in French state institutions.
2. This work developed at the end of the 1990s and through the 2000s with the interdisciplinary research unit Centre de Recherche sur la Santé, le Social et le Politique, which became Institut de Recherche Interdisciplinaire sur les Enjeux Sociaux in 2007. This theme of research also developed at the Unité de Recherche Migration et Société (URMIS) research unit, which focused mainly on immigration and interethnic relations. With URMIS, a research group named Groupe de Recherche Migrations Ethnicité Santé emerged, led by sociologist Marguerite Cognet, to specifically address health inequalities.
3. The practice of entrusting children to family or community members is well documented in sub-Saharan Africa. Therefore, it does "make sense" in local understandings of family ties, even if it implies other motives in the context of immigration and family dispersion.
4. However, during his presidential candidacy speech, Nicolas Sarkozy referred to himself as being French of mixed blood (*un petit français de sang mêlé*) (see *Le Monde* 2007).

4. MANAGING "MIGRANT YOUTH"

Portions of this chapter appeared in another form as part of Larchanché, Stéphanie. 2016. "Health Spaces: Representations of French Immigrant Youth in Mental Health Care." In *Identity and the Second Generation: How Children of Immigrants Find Their Space*, edited by Faith G. Nibbs and Caroline B. Brettell, 172–190. Nashville, TN: Vanderbilt University Press.

1. There is an overall lack of data on this population group because data on ethnicity cannot be collected in the French census or in social science surveys (Simon 2000b). Eventually, in 2010, an exemption was granted to the National Institutes of Statistics and Demographic Studies to carry out the largest survey ever conducted on ethnic minorities in France. This survey produced unique data, particularly on feelings of national belonging ("being French") and "feeling at home" in France (Beauchemin, Hamel, and Simon 2016). The survey was conducted in metropolitan France between September 2008 and February 2009 using a sample of 22,000 people, 8,200 of them representing descendants of migrants.
2. Law of March 18, 2003, on national security (LSI or Loi Sarkozy II): http://www.legifrance .gouv.fr/affichTexte.do?cidTexte=LEGITEXT000005634107&dateTexte=vig.
3. Law of March 5, 2007, on the prevention of delinquency: https://www.legifrance.gouv.fr /affichTexte.do?cidTexte=JORFTEXT000000615568.

4. Reports published in France on employment discrimination are based on candidates' last names (Meurs, Pailhé, and Simon 2006).

5. See my case studies for references to the 2005 law on "handicap" (*Loi n° 2005-102 du 11 février 2005 pour l'égalité des droits et des chances, la participation et la citoyenneté des personnes handicapées*) in France: https://www.legifrance.gouv.fr/affichTexte.do?cidTexte=JORFTEXT 000000809647.

6. ZEPs were created in 1981 (as part of the Mitterand government's social policies) in an effort to address academic failure rates in lower socioeconomic residential areas. In 2006, they were redefined as the Ambition and Success Network. In 2008, they were incorporated into the government's Urban Policy Program (Politique de la ville), the educational agenda of which focuses on "bringing hope back in the suburbs" (*espoir banlieues*). In his inauguration of the program, President Sarkozy pointed out that the "malaise" characterizing French suburbs was not simply related to structural decay but threatened "the very idea of the nation . . . [as] being also related to identity, culture, morality, in short, it is human and not simply material" (Présidence de la République 2008). Since 2014, REPs have replaced ZEPs to include middle schools, but in the national education jargon, the acronym ZEP is still commonly used.

7. RASEDs were created in 1990 by the National Education Ministry as a "resource network," contributing to newly defined politics of school "adaptation and integration."

8. Maître Es and maître Gs receive their training from an Institut universitaires de formation des maîtres (IUFM, National Training Institute for School Teachers). They must already be certified as school teachers and must have at least one year of experience in a regular classroom.

9. Commission des droits et de l'autonomie des personnes handicapées: http://www .travail-solidarite.gouv.fr/spip.php?page=article&id_article=3347.

10. In primary schools, the "pedagogical team" consists of the school director, tenured teachers, replacement teachers, and special aid teachers.

11. The Wechsler Intelligence Scale for Children (WISC), developed by David Wechsler, is an intelligence test for children between the ages of six and sixteen that can be completed without reading or writing and generates an IQ score. The current version, the WISC-IV, was produced in 2003. Each successive version has been reformatted to compensate for the Flynn effect, refining questions to make them less biased against minorities and females. See http://en.wikipedia.org/wiki/Wechsler_Intelligence_Scale_for_Children.

12. School assistants, as mentioned earlier, have an unclear status in schools. The position was created by the government as part of a broader plan to create jobs for the unemployed, and these jobs are usually precarious (short term) and low paid. In schools, the authority of assistants is ill-defined. They are meant to assist teachers in the classroom with students and class activities; however, their role is defined by the teacher or by the school director. For example, they may be required to watch over children during recess, organize school supplies, and undertake other simple tasks.

5. ENACTING CULTURAL COMPETENCE

1. This was the Projet fondation de France #00051304.

6. PSYCHOTHERAPY AT THE BORDERLAND

1. The *M.S.S. case* concerns an Afghan asylum seeker who lodged an asylum application in Belgium. Based on the Dublin II Regulation, Belgium sent him back to Greece, the country through which he had irregularly entered the European Union. In Greece, he was twice placed

in detention, where he was subjected to degrading circumstances. After his release, he was abandoned to live on the streets, without any support from the Greek authorities. Being aware of the structural shortcomings in the asylum procedure and of the systematic problems in the detention and reception of asylum seekers in Greece, the question was whether or not Belgium was allowed to transfer the applicant. These problems were well documented in NGO reports and in international circles, such as the UN High Commissioner for Refugees and the European Committee for the Prevention of Torture. On January 21, 2011, the European Court of Human Rights held that asylum conditions in Greece were so bad that not only Greece but also Belgium had violated the ECHR. Belgium's violation occurred when the government transferred an asylum seeker back to Greece. On September 22, 2011, Verica Trstenjak—advocate general of the European Court of Justice—stated that asylum seekers may not be transferred to other member states if they could there face a risk of serious breach of the fundamental rights that are guaranteed under the Charter of Fundamental Rights.

2. Decree on the questionnaire to detect vulnerabilities among asylum seekers. Available at https://www.legifrance.gouv.fr/eli/arrete/2015/10/23/INTV1523959A/jo.

3. The National Rights Advocate institution (le Défenseur des droits) was created in 2011. It is independent from the state. Its missions are twofold and include defending persons whose rights have not been respected and ensuring equal access to rights for all. It represents the fusion of four different institutions: the Republic's Mediator (le Médiateur de la République), the Children's Ombudsman (le Défenseur des enfants), the High Authority for the Fight against Discrimination and for Equality (la Haute Autorité de lutte contre les discriminations et pour l'égalité) (HALDE), and the National Security Ethics Committee (Commission nationale de déontologie de la sécurité) (CNDS). The report on health-care refusal is available at https://www.defenseurdesdroits.fr/fr/actus/actualites/refus-de-soins-pour-les-beneficiaires -de-protection-sociale-cmuacsame-le-defenseur.

4. Because of their special needs, the health-care system dispenses with CMU and AME patients paying their consultation fee up front, which means that doctors are paid only when the social security system processes the claim and reimburses them.

7. BEYOND ANXIETIES: PRAXIS

1. Médecins et patients face aux maladies chroniques: Quelle alliance? Une approche transculturelle, October 23, 2013, City Hall, Paris.

2. Concilier valeurs hospitalières et contraintes économiques: un enjeu majeur pour un système de santé en évolution, November 21, 2017, Ministry of Health and Solidarity, Paris.

REFERENCES

Agier, Michel. 2013. *La condition cosmopolite: L'anthropologie à l'épreuve du piège identitaire*. Paris: La Découverte.

———. 2016. *Les migrants et nous: Comprendre Babel*. Paris: CNRS Editions.

———. 2017. "Définir les réfugiés? La demande d'asile en mots et en situation: Entretien avec Anne-Virginie Madeira." In *Définir les réfugiés*, edited by Michel Agier and Anne-Virginie Madeira, 9–27. Paris: Presses Universitaires de France.

Akoka, Karen. 2017. "Distinguer les réfugiés des migrants au XXe siècle: Enjeux et usages des politiques de classification." In *Définir les réfugiés*, edited by Michel Agier and Anne-Virginie Madeira, 47–68. Paris: Presses Universitaires de France.

Alliez, Joseph, and Henri Descombes. 1952. "Réflexions sur le comportement psycho-pathologique d'une série de nord-africains musulmans immigrés." *Annales médico-psychologiques* 110 (2): 150–156.

Andoche, Jacqueline. 2001. "Santé Mentale et Culture: Les Avatars Français de l'Ethnopsychiatrie." In *Critique de la santé publique: Une approche anthropologique*, edited by Jean-Pierre Dozon and Didier Fassin, 281–308. Paris: Balland.

Ansari, David. 2014. "Cultural Expertise and Triage: Context, Mediation, and Treatment Management in Psychiatric Services in Paris." Master's thesis, University of Chicago.

Asad, Talal, ed. 1973. *Anthropology and the Colonial Encounter*. New York: Humanities Press.

Association Françoise et Eugène Minkowski. 2017. *Rapport d'activité 2016*.

Barou, Jacques. 1999. "Trajectoires residentielles, du bidobville au logement social." In *Immigration et intégration, l'état des savoirs*, edited by Philippe Dewitte, 185–195. Paris: La Découverte.

———. 2002. "Les immigrations africaines en France au tournant du siècle." In "Africains, citoyens d'ici et de là-bas." *Hommes et migrations* 1239:6–18.

Baubet, Thierry, Tahar Abbal, Catherine Le Du, Felicia Heidenreich, Katherine Lévy, Sahim Mehallel, Dalila Rezzoug, Gesine Sturm, and Marie Rose Moro. 2004. "Traumas psychiques chez les demandeurs d'asile en France: Des spécificités cliniques et thérapeutiques." In *Le journal international de victimologie* 2 (2).

Beauchemin, Cris, Christelle Hamel, and Patrick Simon. 2016. *Trajectoires et origines: Enquête sur la diversité des populations en France*. Paris: INED.

Beck, Ulrich, Anthony Giddens, and Scott Lash. 1994. *Reflexive Modernization: Politics, Tradition and Aesthetics in the Modern Social Order*. Cambridge: Polity Press.

Beneduce, Roberto. 2006. "L'apport de Frantz Fanon à l'ethnopsychiatrie critique. " In *VST - Vie sociale et traitements* 89 (1): 85–100.

———. 2016. "Traumatic Pasts and the Historical Imagination: Symptoms of Loss, Postcolonial Suffering, and Counter-Memories among African Migrants." In *Transcultural Psychiatry* 53 (3): 261–285.

Bénisti, Jacques Alain. 2005. *Sur la prévention de la délinquance: Rapport préliminaire de la commission prévention du groupe d'études parlementaire sur la sécurité intérieure*. October 2005. http://38.snuipp.fr/IMG/pdf/rapport_BENISTI_prevention.pdf.

Benjamin, Ilil. 2015. "Medical NGOs in Strong States: Working the Margins of the Israeli Medical Bureaucracy." In *Medical Humanitarianism: Ethnographies of Practice*, edited by

Sharon Abramowitz and Catherine Panter-Brick, 226–241. Philadelphia: University of Pennsylvania Press.

Bennani, Jalil. (1980) 2015. *Le corps suspect: Le corps du migrant face à l'institution médicale.* Paris: La Croisée Des Chemins.

Bennegadi, Rachid. 1996. "Anthropologie médicale clinique et santé mentale des migrants en France." In *Médecine tropicale: Revue française de pathologie et de santé publique tropicales* 56 (4): 445–452.

Benoit de Coignac, Agathe, and Thierry Baubet. 2013. "Transes et construction identitaire chez les mineurs isolés étrangers." In *Adolescence* 31 (3): 613–623. https://doi.org/10.3917/ado.085.0613.

Benslama, Fethi. 1996. "L'illusion ethnopsychiatrique." *Le Monde*, December 4, 1996.

———. 2004. "Qu'est-ce qu'une clinique de l'exil?" In *L'Evolution Psychiatrique* 69 (1): 23–30.

Bernardot, Marc. 2008. "Camps d'étrangers, foyers de travailleurs, centres d'expulsion: Les lieux communs de l'immigré décolonisé." *Cultures et conflits* 69: 55–79.

Bertossi, Christophe, and Catherine Wihtol de Wenden. 2007. *Les couleurs du Drapeau: L'armée française face aux discriminations.* Paris: Robert Laffont.

Biehl, João. 2005. *Vita: Life in a Zone of Social Abandonment.* Berkeley: University of California Press.

Boltanski, Luc. 1999. *Distant Suffering: Politics, Morality and the Media.* Cambridge: Cambridge University Press.

Bouquet, Brigitte. 2006. "Management et travail social." *Revue française de gestion* 168–169 (9): 125–141.

Bourdieu, Pierre. 1977. *Outline of a Theory of Practice.* Cambridge: Cambridge University Press.

———. 1991. *Language and Symbolic Power.* Cambridge, MA: Harvard University Press.

———. 1996. "Prologue: Social Structures and Mental Structures." In *The State Nobility: Elite Schools in the Field of Power*, translated by Lauretta C. Oxford: Polity Press.

Bourdieu, Pierre, Alain Accardo, Gabrielle Balazs, Stephane Beaud, François Bonvin, Emmanuel Bourdieu, Philippe Bourgois, et al. 1999. *The Weight of the World: Social Suffering in Contemporary Society.* Translated by Pricilla Parkhurst Ferguson, Susan Emanuel, Joe Johnson, and Shoggy T. Waryn. Stanford, CA: Stanford University Press.

Bourdin, Marie-Jo. 2006. *L'excision, une coutume à l'épreuve de la loi.* Ivry-su-Seine: A3.

———. 2013. *Les blanches ne sont pas frigides: Traumatisme-Excision-Normes de la sexualité.* Editions Panafrica/Nouvelles du Sud.

Bouznah, Serge, and Catherine Lewertowski. 2013. *Quand les esprits viennent aux médecins: 7 récits pour soigner.* Paris: In press.

Bowen, John. 2007. *Why the French Don't Like Headscarves: Islam, the State, and Public Space.* Princeton, NJ: Princeton University Press.

Bricaud, Julien. 2006. *Mineurs isolés étrangers: L'épreuve du soupçon.* Paris: Vuibert.

Briggs, Charles. 2005. "Communicability, Racial Discourse, and Disease." In *Annual Review of Anthropology* 34: 269–291.

Brinbaum, Yaël, Dominique Meurs, and Jean-Luc Primon. 2015. "Situation sur la marche du travail: statuts d'activité, accès à l'emploi, et discrimination." In *Trajectoires et origines: Enquête sur la diversité des populations en France*, 203–232. Paris: Ined.

Brinbaum, Yaël, and Jean-Luc Primon. 2013. "Parcours scolaires et sentiment d'injustice et de discrimination chez les descendants d'immigrés." In *Economie et statistique* 464-465-466:215–243. https://www.insee.fr/fr/statistiques/fichier/1378029/ES464M.pdf.

Brodwin, Paul. 2013. *Everyday Ethics: Voices from the Frontline of Community Psychiatry.* Berkeley: University of California Press.

Capogna-Bardet, Ghislaine, ed. 2014. *La clinique du trauma.* Ers: Collection Centre Primo Levi.

Carde, Estelle. 2006. "Les discriminations selon l'origine dans l'accès aux soins: Etude en France métropolitaine et en Guyane française." PhD diss., Université Paris XI.

Carde, Estelle, Didier Fassin, Nathalie Ferré, and Sandrine Musso-Dimitrijevic. 2002. "Un traitement inégal: Les dicriminations dans l'accès aux soins." *Migrations études* 106: 1–12.

Carlin, Maria Vittoria. 2017. "Questions autour de la prise en charge des personnes réfugiées: Temps, récit traumatique et relation thérapeutique. Diplôme Universitaire 'Psychopathologie et psychotraumatisme.'" Thesis, Université Paris Diderot.

Carpenter-Song, Elizabeth A., Megan Nordquest Schwallie, and Jeffrey Longhofer. 2007. "Cultural Competence Reexamined: Critique and Directions for the Future." In *Psychiatric Services* 58: 1362–1365.

Casadesus, Frédérick. "Migrants, politique migratoire et intégration: Le constat d'Emmanuel Macron." *Réforme*, March 2, 2017.

Castañeda, Heide. 2010. "Im/Migration and Health: Conceptual, Methodological, and Theoretical Propositions for Applied Anthropology." *NAPA Bulletin* 34 (1): 6–27.

Castañeda, Heide, Seth M. Holmes, Daniel S. Madrigal, Maria-Elena De Trinidad Young, Naomi Beyeler, and James Quesada. 2015. "Immigration as a Social Determinant of Health." In *Annual Review of Public Health* 36:375–392.

Cediey, Eric, and Fabrice Foroni. 2008. *Discrimination in Access to Employment on Grounds of Foreign Origin in France: A National Survey of Discrimination Based on the Testing Methodology of the International Labour Office*. Geneva: International Labour Office, International Migration Programme. https://www.ilo.org/wcmsp5/groups/public/---ed_protect/---protrav/---migrant/documents/publication/wcms_201429.pdf.

Chambon, Nicolas. 2013. "Le migrant précaire comme nouvelle figure du débordement." *Rhizome* 48:5–6.

———. 2017. "Migration et santé mentale, quelles perspectives depolitisation?" *Rhizome* 1 (63): 90–97.

Chambon, Nicolas, and Gwen Le Goff. 2016. "Enjeux et controverses de la prise en charge des migrants précaires en psychiatrie." *Revue française des affaires sociales* 2 (6): 123–140.

Charte MCS. 2006. *Charte de la Médiation Sociale et Culturelle dans les Hauts-de-Seine*. Paris: Département des Hauts-de-Seine.

Clifford, James, and George E. Marcus. 1986. *Writing Culture. The Poetics and Politics of Ethnography*. Berkeley: University of California Press.

Codó, Eva. 2008. *Immigration and Bureaucratic Control: Language Practices in Public Administration*. Berlin: Walter de Gruyter.

Cognet, Marguerite. 2007. "Au nom de la culture: Le recours à la culture dans la santé." In *Ethique de l'altérité: La question de la culture dans la santé et les services sociaux*, edited by Marguerite Cognet and Catherine Montgomery, 39–63. Québec: Presses de l'Université Laval.

Comaroff, Jean. 1985. *Body of Power, Spirit of Resistance: The Culture and History of a South African People*. Chicago: University of Chicago Press.

———. 1993. "Diseased Heart of Africa. Medicine, Colonialism, and the Black Body." In *Knowledge, Power and Practice: The Anthropology of Medicine and Everyday Life*, edited by Shirley Lindenbaum and Margaret Lock, 305–329. Berkeley: University of California Press.

Copping, Alicia, Jane Shakespeare-Finch, and Douglas Paton. 2010. "Towards a Culturally Appropriate Mental Health System: Sudanese-Australians' Experiences with Trauma." *Journal of Pacific Rim Psychology* 4 (1): 53–60.

Coutant, Isabelle, and Jean-Sébastien Eideliman. 2013. "À l'écoute des souffrances: Fragilité psychique et fragilité sociale dans une maison des adolescents." In *Juger, réprimer, accompagner: Essai sur la morale de l'état*, edited by Didier Fassin, Yasmine Bouagga, Isabelle

Coutant, Jean-Sébastien Eideliman, Fabrice Fernandez, Nicolas Fischer, Carolina Kobelinsky, Chowra Makaremi, Sarah Mazouz, and Sébastien Roux, 271–308. Paris: Le Seuil.

Crenn, Chantal, and Laurence Kotobi, eds. 2012. *Du point de vue de l'ethnicité, pratiques françaises*. Paris: Armand Colin.

CSA. 2014. *Représentations de la diversité de la société française à la télévision et à la radio: Rapport au Parlement*. Avril 2014.

Csordas, Thomas J. 1994. *Embodiment and Experience: The Existential Ground of Culture and Self*. New York: Cambridge University Press.

d'Albis, Hippolyte, and Ekrame Boubtane. 2018. "L'admission au séjour des demandeurs d'asile en France depuis 2000." *Population et Sociétés* 552. https://www.ined.fr/fichier/s_rubrique /27442/pop.soc_552.migration.asile.fr.pdf.

Dahoun, Salima Zerdalia. 1992. "Les us et abus de l'ethnopsychiatrie: Le patient migrant; Sujet souffrant ou objet d'expérimentation clinique?" *Les temps modernes* 552–553: 223–251.

Das, Veena. 2001. *Remaking a World: Violence, Social Suffering, and Recovery*. Berkeley: University of California Press.

Das, Veena, Arthur Kleinman, Margaret Lock, Mamphela Ramphele, and Pamela Reynolds, eds. 2000. *Violence and Subjectivity*. Berkeley: University of California Press.

Daum, Christophe. 1998. *Les associations de Maliens en France: Migration, développement, et citoyenneté*. Paris: Karthala.

De Rudder, Véronique. 1999. "Jalons pour une histoire sociopolitique de la recherche sur les relations interethniques en France." In *Migrations internationales et relations interethniques, recherche politique et société*, edited by I. R. Barouch and V. De Rudder, 74–96. Paris: L'Harmattan.

DelVecchio Good, Mary-Jo, Cara James, Byron Good, and Anne Becker. 2003. "The Culture of Medicine and Racial, Ethnic, and Class Disparities in Health Care." In *Unequal Treatment: Confronting Racial and Ethnic Disparities in Health Care*, edited by Brian D. Smedley, Adrienne Y. Stith, and Alan R. Nelson, 594–625. Washington, D.C.: IOM, National Academies Press.

DelVecchio Good, Mary-Jo, Sarah S. Willen, Seth Donal Hannah, Ken Vickery, and Lawrence Taeseng Park, eds. 2011. *Shattering Culture: American Medicine Responds to Cultural Diversity*. New York: Russell Sage Foundation.

Derrida, Jacques, and Anne Dufourmantelle. 1997. *De l'hospitalité*. Paris: Calmann-Lévy.

Desjarlais, Robert R. 1992. *Body and Emotion: The Aesthetics of Illness and Healing in the Nepal Himalayas*. Philadelphia: University of Pennsylvania Press.

Desprès, Caroline, and Pierre Lombrail. 2017. *Résultats de l'étude: "Des pratiques médicales et dentaires, entre différenciation et discrimination." Une analyse du discours des médecins et dentistes*. https://www.defenseurdesdroits.fr/sites/default/files/atoms/files/etudesresultats-oit -03.04.17-num-final.pdf.

Devereux, George. 1967. *From Anxiety to Method in the Behavioral Sciences*. The Hague: Mouton.

———. 1970. *Essais d'ethnopsychiatrie générale*. Paris: Bibliothèque des Sciences Humaines.

———. 1980. *Basic Problems of Ethnopsychiatry*. Chicago: University of Chicago Press.

d'Halluin, Estelle. 2009. "La santé mentale des demandeurs d'asile." In "Santé et droits des étrangers: Réalités et enjeux." *Hommes et migrations* 1282: 66–75.

d'Halluin-Mabillot, Estelle. 2012. *Les épreuves de l'asile: Associations et réfugiés face aux politiques du soupçon*. Paris: EHESS.

Dhume, Fabrice, Suzana Dukic, Séverine Chauvel and Philippe Perrot. 2011. *Orientation scolaire et discrimination. De l'(in)égalité de traitement selon "l'origine."* Paris : La Documentation française.

Dominicé Dao, Melissa, Sophie Inglin, Sarah Vilpert, and Patricia Hudelson. 2018. "The Relevance of Clinical Ethnography: Reflections on 10 Years of a Cultural Consultation Service." *BMC Health Services Research* 18 (19). https://bmchealthservres.biomedcentral.com/track/pdf/10.1186/s12913-017-2823-x.

Douville, Olivier, and Laurent Ottavi. 1995. "Champ anthropologique et clinique du sujet: Exemples des cliniques de la transmission dans l'exil." *Migrants formation* 103.

Dubet, François. 2004. *L'école des chances: Qu'est-ce qu'une école juste?* Paris: Seuil.

Dubet François, Olivier Cousin, Eric Macé and Sandrine Rui. 2013. *Pourquoi moi? L'expérience des discriminations.* Paris: Seuil.

Dubet, François, and Danilo Martucelli. 1996. *A l'école: Sociologie de l'expérience scolaire.* Paris: Seuil.

Durkheim, Emile. (1914) 1973. "The Dualism of Human Nature and Its Social Conditions." In *Emile Durkheim on Morality and Society,* edited by Robert N. Bellah, 149–167. Chicago: University of Chicago Press.

Durkheim, Emile, and Marcel Mauss. 1963. *Primitive Classification.* Translated and edited with an introduction by Rodney Needham. Chicago: University of Chicago Press.

Durpaire, François. 2006. *France blanche, colère noire.* Paris: Odile Jacob.

Essed, Philomena. 1991. *Understanding Everyday Racism: An Interdisciplinary Theory.* Newbury Park, CA: Sage.

Etiemble, Angélina, and Omar Zanna. 2013. "Des typologies pour faire connaissance avec les mineurs isolés étrangers et mieux les accompagner." In *Synthèse de la Convention de recherche n°212.01.09.14: "Actualiser et complexifier la typologie des motifs de départ du pays d'origine des mineurs isolés étrangers présents en France." Topik/Mission de Recherche Droit et Justice.* https://infomie.net/IMG/pdf/synthese_-_actualisation_typologie_mie_2013-2.pdf.

European Court of Human Rights. 2011. *Arrêt M.S.S. c. Belgique et Grèce,* no. 30696/09. January 21. http://www.gdr-elsj.eu/wp-content/uploads/2017/02/AFFAIRE-M.S.S.-c.-BELGIQUE-ET-GRECE-1.pdf.

Fadiman, Anne. 1997. *The Spirit Catches You and You Fall Down: A Hmong Child, Her American Doctors, and the Collision of Two Cultures.* New York: Farrar, Straus and Giroux.

Fanon, Frantz. 1952. "Le 'syndrome nord-africain.'" *Esprit,* February 1952, 237–285.

———. 1973. *The Wretched of the Earth,* 2nd ed. New York: Ballantine.

Fanon, Frantz, and Jacques Azoulay. 1954. "La socialthérapie dans un service d'hommes musulmans: Difficultés méthodologiques." In *L'information psychiatrique* 30 (9): 349–361.

Fargues, Philippe. 2016. "Who Are the Million Migrants Who Entered Europe without a Visa in 2015? *Population et Sociétés* 532. https://www.ined.fr/fichier/s_rubrique/25200/532.population.and.societies.april.2016.eng.migration.europe.en.pdf.

Farmer, Paul. 1996. "On Suffering and Structural Violence: A View from Below." *Daedalus* 125 (1): 261–283.

———. 2004. "An Anthropology of Structural Violence." *Current Anthropology* 45:305–326.

Farmer, Paul E., Bruce Nizeye, Sara Stulac, Salmaan Keshavjee. 2006. "Structural Violence and Clinical Medicine." *PLoS Med* 3 (10): e449. https://doi.org/10.1371/journal.pmed.0030449.

Fassin, Didier. 1999. "L'ethnopsychiatrie et ses reseaux: L'influence qui grandit." *Genèses* 35: 146–171.

———. 2000. "Les politiques de l'ethnopsychiatrie: La psyché africaine, des colonies africaines aux banlieues parisiennes." *L'Homme* 153: 231–250.

———. 2001. "The Biopolitics of Otherness: Undocumented Foreigners and Racial Undocumented Foreigners and Racial Discrimination in French Public Debate." *Anthropology Today* 17 (1): 3–7.

———. 2004. *Des maux indicibles: Sociologie des lieux d'écoute*. Paris: La Découverte.

———. 2005. "Compassion and Repression: The Moral Economy of Immigration Policies in France." *Cultural Anthropology* 20 (3): 362–387.

———. 2006. "Nommer, interpreter: Le sens commun de la question raciale." *De la question sociale à la question raciale? Représenter la société française*. Paris: La Découverte.

———. 2012. "Introduction: Toward a Critical Moral Anthropology." In *A Companion to Moral Anthropology*, edited by Didier Fassin, 1–17. Malden: Wiley-Blackwell.

Fassin, Didier, Yasmine Bouagga, Isabelle Coutant, Jean-Sébastien Eideliman, Fabrice Fernandez, Nicolas Fischer, Carolina Kobelinsky, Chowra Makaremi, Sarah Mazouz, and Sébastien Roux. 2013. *Juger, réprimer, accompagner: Essai sur la morale de l'état*. Paris: Editions du Seuil.

Fassin, Didier, and Estelle d'Halluin. 2005. "The Truth from the Body: Medical Certificates as Ultimate Evidence for Asylum Seekers." In *American Anthropologist* 107 (4): 597–608.

Fassin, Didier, and Jean-Pierre Dozon, eds. 2001. *Critique de la santé publique: Une approche anthropologique*. Paris: Balland.

Fassin, Didier, and Eric Fassin, eds. 2009. *De la question sociale à la question raciale? Représenter la société française*, 2nd ed. Paris: La Découverte/Poche.

Fassin, Didier, Alain Morice, and Catherine Quiminal. 1997. *Les lois de l'inhospitalité: Les politiques de l'immigration à l'épreuve des sans papiers*. Paris: La Découverte.

Fassin, Didier, and Anne-Jeanne Naudé. 2004. "Plumbism Reinvented: Childhood Lead Poisoning in France, 1985–1990." *American Journal of Public Health* 94 (11): 1854–1863.

Fassin, Didier, and Richard Rechtman. 2005. "An Anthropological Hybrid: The Pragmatic Arrangement of Universalism and Culturalism in French Mental Health." *Transcultural Psychiatry* 42 (3): 347–366.

———. 2009. *The Empire of Trauma: An Inquiry into the Condition of Victimhood*. Princeton, NJ: Princeton University Press.

Felouzis, Georges, Joëlle Favre-Perroton, and Françoise Liot. 2005. *L'Apartheid scolaire: Enquête sur la ségrégation ethnique dans les collèges*. Paris: Seuil.

Felouzis, Georges, and Barbara Fouquet-Chauprade, eds. 2015. "Les descendants d'immigrés à l'école: Destins scolaires et origines des inégalités." Special issue, *Revue française de pédagogie* 191. https://rfp.revues.org/4735.

Foucault, Michel. (1963) 1994. *The Birth of the Clinic: An Archeology of Medical Perception*. New York: Vintage Books.

Freud, Sigmund. (1949) 1989. *An Outline of Psychoanalysis*, edited by James Strachey, with an introduction by Peter Gay. New York: W. W. Norton.

Furtos, Jean, ed. 2008. *Les cliniques de la précarité: Contexte sociale, psychopathologie et dispositifs*. Paris: Elsevier Masson.

Gaines, Atwood. 1992. "From DSM-I to III-R: Voices of Self, Mastery, and the Other; A Cultural Constructivist Reading of US Psychiatric Classification." *Social Science and Medicine* 35: 3–24.

Garcia, Angela. 2010. *The Pastoral Clinic: Addiction and Dispossession along the Rio Grande*. Los Angeles: University of California Press.

Gaspar, Jean-François. 2012. *Tenir! Les raisons d'être des travailleurs sociaux*. Paris: La Découverte.

Georges-Tarragano, Claire, Christine Girier-Debolt, and Lucie Davakan-Alonso. 2017. "Ethique de gestion et valeur du soin. Des enjeux pluri professionnels." *Journal de l'association des directeurs d'hôpital* 72.

Gilloire, Augustin. 2000. "Les catégories d''origine' et de 'nationalité' dans les statistiques du sida." In "Santé: Le traitement de la différence." *Hommes et migrations* 1225:73–82.

Giordano, Cristiana. 2014. *Migrants in Translation: Caring and the Logics of Difference in Contemporary Italy.* Berkeley: University of California Press.

Goguikian Ratcliff, Betty. 2012. "Repenser les liens entre migration, exil et traumatisme." *(Re)penser l'exil* 1 (February). https://archive-ouverte.unige.ch/files/downloads/0/0/0/3/4/3/2/0/unige_34320_attachment01.pdf.

Good, Byron, and Mary-Jo DelVecchio Good. 1993. "'Learning Medicine': The Constructing of Medical Knowledge at Harvard Medical School." In *Knowledge, Power, and Practice: The Anthropology of Medicine and Everyday Life,* edited by Shirley Lindenbaum and Margaret Lock, 81–108. Berkeley: University of California Press.

———. 2010. "Amok in Java: Madness and violence in Indonesian politics." In *A reader in medical anthropology: Theoretical trajectories, emergent realities,* edited by Byron J. Good, Michael M. J. Fischer, Sarah S. Willen, and Mary-Jo DelVecchio Good, 473–480. Malden, MA: Wiley-Blackwell.

Goris, Indira, Fabien Jobard, and René Lévy. 2009. *Profiling Minorities: A Study of Stop-and-Search Practices in Paris.* New York: Open Society Institute.

Granger, Bernard, ed. 1999. *Eugène Minkowski: Une oeuvre philosphique, psychiatrique, et sociale.* Levallois-Perret: Editions Interligne.

Guarnaccia, Peter. 2003. "Editorial. Methodological advances in cross-cultural study of mental health: setting new standards." *Culture, Medicine and Psychiatry* 27 (3): 249–257.

Guzder, Jaswant, and Cécile Rousseau. 2013. "A Diversity of Voices: The McGill 'Working with Culture' Seminars." *Culture, Medicine and Psychiatry* 37 (2): 347–364.

Haas, Bridget M. 2017. "Citizens-in-Waiting, Deportees-in-Waiting: Power, Temporality, and Suffering in the US Asylum System." *Ethos* 45 (1): 75–97.

Hansen, Helena, Joel Braslow, and Robert M. Rohrbaugh. 2018. "From Cultural to Structural Competency: Training Psychiatry Residents to Act on Social Determinants of Health and Institutional Racism." *JAMA Psychiatry* 75 (2): 117–118.

Hargreaves, Alec G. 1995. *Immigration, "Race" and Ethnicity in Contemporary France.* New York: Routledge.

HAS. 2017. "Historique de la certification." June 8. https://www.has-sante.fr/portail/jcms/c_978601/fr/historique-de-la-certification.

Héran, François. 2017. *Avec l'immigration. Mesurer, débattre, agir.* Paris, La Découverte.

Holmes, Seth M., and Heide Castañeda. 2016. "Representing the 'European Refugee Crisis' in Germany and Beyond: Deservingness and Difference, Life and Death." *American Ethnologist,* 43(1): 12–24.

Hughes, Charles. 1996. "Ethnopsychiatry." In *Medical Anthropology: Contemporary Theory and Method,* edited by Thomas M. Johnson and Carolyn F. Sargent, 131–151. Westport, CT: Praeger.

Hunt, Nancy Rose. 1999. *A Colonial Lexicon of Birth Ritual, Medicalization, and Mobility in the Congo.* Durham, NC: Duke University Press.

Ichou, Mathieu. 2013. "Différences d'origine et origine des différences: Les résultats scolaires des enfants d'émigrés/immigrés en France du début de l'école primaire à la fin du collège." *Revue française de sociologie* 54 (1): 5–52.

Ichou, Mathieu, and Agnès van Zanten. 2014. "France." In *The Palgrave Handbook of Race and Ethnic Inequalities in Education,* edited by Peter A. Stevens and A. Gary Dworkin, 328–364. New York: Palgrave Macmillan.

Idris, Isam. 2009. "Cultures, migration et sociétés : destin des loyautés familiales et culturelles chez les enfants de migrants. " *Dialogue* 184 (2), 131–140.

Irvine, Judith T., and Susan Gal. 2000. "Language Ideology and Linguistic Differentiation." In *Regimes of Language: Ideologies, Polities, and Identities,* edited by P. V. Kroskrity, 35–84. Santa Fe: School of American Research Press.

Izambert, Caroline. 2016. "Logiques de tri et discriminations à l'hôpital public: Vers une nouvelle morale hospitalière?" *Agone* 1 (58): 89–104.

Jacques, Paul. 2004. "Souffrance psychique et souffrance sociale." *Pensée Plurielle* 2 (8): 21–29.

Jenkins, Janis H. 1991. "Anthropology, Expressed Emotion, and Schizophrenia." *Ethos* 19 (4): 387–431.

———. 1996. "Culture, Emotion, and Psychiatric Distress." In *Handbook of Medical Anthropology: Cotemporary Theory and Method*, edited by Carolyn F. Sargent and Thomas M. Johnson, 71–87. Westport, CT: Greenwood Press.

Jenkins, Janis H., and Robert J. Barrett. 2004. *Schizophrenia, Culture, and Subjectivity: The Edge of Experience*. New York: Cambridge University Press.

Keller, Richard C. 2007. "Between Clinical and Useful Knowledge: Race, Ethnicity, and the Conquest of the Primitive." *Colonial Madness: Psychiatry in French North Africa*, 121–160. Chicago: University of Chicago Press.

Kirmayer, Laurence J. 1997. "Somatization in Social and Cultural Perspective: From Research to Clinical Strategies." *Japanese Journal of Psychosomatic Medicine* 37 (6): 311–319.

———. 2008. "Empathy and Alterity in Cultural Psychiatry." *Ethos* 36 (4): 457–474.

———. 2012. "Rethinking Cultural Competence." *Transcultural Psychiatry* 49 (2): 149–164.

———. 2013. "Embracing Uncertainty as a Path to Competence: Cultural Safety, Empathy, and Alterity in Clinical Training." *Cult Med Psychiatry* 37: 365–372.

Kirmayer, Laurence, Hannah Kienzler, Abdel Hamid Afana, and Duncan Pedersen. 2010. "Trauma and Disasters in Social and Cultural Context." In *Principles of Social Psychiatry*, 2nd ed., edited by Craig Morgan and Dinesh Bhugra, 155–177. Chichester, UK: Wiley-Blackwell.

Kirmayer, Laurence, Jaswant Guzder, and Cécile Rousseau, eds. 2014. *Cultural Consultation Encountering the Other in Mental Health Care*. New York: Springer.

Kirmayer, Laurence J., Rachel Kronick, and Cécile Rousseau. 2018. "Advocacy as Key to Structural Competency in Psychiatry." *JAMA Psychiatry* 75 (2): 119–120.

Kleinman, Arthur. 1980. *Patients and Healers in the Context of Culture: An Exploration of the Borderland between Anthropology, Medicine, and Psychiatry*. Berkeley, CA: University of California.

———. 1988. *The Illness Narratives: Suffering, Healing, and the Human Condition*. New York: Basic Books.

———. 2012. "The Art of Medicine: Caregiving as a Moral Experience." *Lancet* 380:1550–1551.

Kleinman, Arthur, and Pete Benson. 2006. "Anthropology in the Clinic: The Problem of Cultural Competency and How to Fix It." *PLoS Medicine* 3: 1673–1676.

Kleinman, Arthur, Veena Das, and Margaret Lock, eds. 1997. *Social Suffering*. Berkeley: University of California Press.

Kleinman, Arthur, Leon Eisenberg, and Byron Good. 1978. "Culture, Illness, and Care: Clinical Lessons from Anthropological and Cross-Cultural Research." *Annals of Internal Medicine* 88 (2): 251–258.

Kleinman, Arthur, and Byron Good, eds. 1985. *Culture and Depression: Studies in Anthropology and Cross-Cultural Psychiatry of Affect and Disorder*. Los Angeles: University of California Press.

Kleinman, Julie. 2016. "'All Daughters and Sons of the Republic'? Producing Difference in French Education." *Journal of the Royal Anthropological Institute* 22: 261–278.

Kohrt, Brandon A., and Emily Mendenhall, eds. 2015. *Global Mental Health: Anthropological Perspectives*. New York: Routledge.

Kotobi, Laurence. 2000. "Le malade dans sa différence: Les professionnels et les patients migrants africains à l'hôpital." In "Santé: Le traitement de la différence." *Hommes et migrations* 1225: 62–72.

Kotobi, Laurence, Stéphanie Larchanché, and Zahia Kessar. 2013. "Enjeux et logiques du recours à l'interprétariat en milieu hospitalier: Une recherche-action autour de l'annonce." In "Les soignants face aux migrants: Représentations et pratiques cliniques," edited by Marguerite Cognet and Priscille Sauvegrain. Special issue, *Migrations Santé* 146–147:53–80.

Laforcade, Michel. 2016. *Rapport relatif à la santé mentale: Ministère des Affaires Sociales et de la Santé.* http://solidarites-sante.gouv.fr/IMG/pdf/dgos_rapport_laforcade_mission_sante_mentale_011016.pdf.

Lamont, Michèle. 2000. *The Dignity of Working Men: Morality and the Boundaries of Race, Class, and Immigration.* Cambridge, MA: Harvard University Press.

Larchanché, Stéphanie. 2010. *Cultural Anxieties and Institutional Regulation: "Specialized" Mental Healthcare and "Immigrant Suffering" in Paris, France.* PhD diss., Washington University in St. Louis and EHESS, Paris.

———. 2012. "Intangible Obstacles: Health Implications of Stigmatization, Structural Violence, and Fear among Undocumented Immigrants in France." In "Migration, 'Illegality,' and Health: Mapping Vulnerability and Debating 'Deservingness,'" edited by Sarah Willen. Special issue, *Social Science and Medicine* 74 (6): 858–863.

Latour, Bruno, and Isabelle Stengers. 1997. "Du bon usage de l'ethnopsychiatrie." *Libération,* January 21, 1997.

Le Blanc, Guillaume, and Fabienne Brugère. 2017. *La fin de l'hospitalité. Lampedusa, Lesbos, Calais . . . jusqu'où irons-nous?* Paris: Flammarion.

Le Figaro. 2015. "La Drôme ne veut plus faire appel à des interprètes dans ses centres médico-sociaux." http://www.lefigaro.fr/actualite-france/2015/10/27/01016-20151027ARTFIG00360-centres-medico-sociaux-la-drome-ne-veut-plus-faire-appel-a-des-interpretes.php.

Le Goaziou, Véronique, and Laurent Muchielli, eds. 2006. *Quand les banlieues brûlent: Retour sur les émeutes de novembre 2005.* Paris: La Découverte.

Le Monde. 2005. "Nicolas Sarkozy fixe un objectif de 25 000 immigrés en situation irrégulière expulsés en 2006." November 29, 2005.

———. 2006. "Regroupement familial et polygamie au banc des accusés." October 23, 2006.

———. 2007. "Le discours d'investiture de Nicolas Sarkozy." January 15, 2007.

———. 2017. "Collomb veut 'distinguer le droit d'asile des autres motifs de migration.'" August 6, 2017. http://www.lemonde.fr/politique/article/2017/08/06/collomb-veut-distinguer-le-droit-d-asile-et-les-autres-motifs-de-migrations_5169204_823448.html#WcGqOJmubKD0GOQd.99.

Levinas, Emmanuel. (1961) 1991. *Totalité et infini: Essai sur l'extériorité.* Paris: Le livre de poche.

Lévy-Bruhl, Lucien. 1923. *Primitive Mentality,* translated by Lilian A. Clare. London: George Allen and Unwin.

L'Express. 2015. "La situation sanitaire des migrants de Calais est pire que dans les pays en guerre." October 21, 2015.

L'Humanité. 1991. "Porteurs de haine." June 21, 1991. https://www.humanite.fr/node/23833.

Lock, Margaret, and Nancy Scheper-Hughes. 1996. "A Critical-Interpretive Approach in Medical Anthropology: Rituals of Discipline and Dissent." *Medical Anthropology: Contemporary Theory and Method,* edited by Carolyn F. Sargent and Thomas M. Johnson, 41–70. Westport, CT: Praeger.

Lorcerie, Françoise. 2011. "École et ethnicité en France: Pour une approche systémique contextualisée." *SociologieS.* October 18, 2011. http://sociologies.revues.org/3706.

Lutz, Catherine, and Geoffrey M. White. 1986. "The Anthropology of Emotions." *Annual Review of Anthropology* 15: 405–436.

Mahyeux, D., ed. 2017. "Adolescence en exil: les parcours pluriels et singuliers des mineurs non accompagnés: Récits, réflexions et pratiques autour d'une situation paradoxale." Special issue, *Revue de l'enfance et de l'adolescence* 96 (2).

Mannoni, Octave. 1950. *Prospero and Caliban: The Psychology of Colonization.* New York: Praeger.

Muni Toke, Valelia. 2009. "Fantasmes d'un plurilinguisme pathogène : le cas des rapports dits 'bénisti'". *Le français aujourd'hui,* 164 (1): 35–44.

Mars, Louis. 1953. "Introduction à l'ethnopsychiatrie." *Bulletin de l'Association Médicale Haïtienne* 6 (2).

Masquet, Brigitte. 2006. "Politique de l'immigration." *Regards sur l'actualité* 326.

Mbembe, Achille. 2013. *Critique de la raison nègre.* Paris: La Découverte.

———. 2016. *Politiques de l'inimitié.* Paris: La Découverte.

McCulloch, Jock. 1995. *Colonial Psychiatry and the "African Mind."* Cambridge: Cambridge University Press.

Médecins du Monde. 2016. *Rapport de l'observatoire de l'accès aux droits et aux soins en France en 2016.* https://www.medecinsdumonde.org/fr/actualites/publications/2017/10/13/rapport-de-lobservatoire-de-lacces-aux-droits-et-aux-soins-en-france-2016.

Mehan, Hugh. 1996. "The Construction of an LD Student." In *Natural Histories of Discourse,* edited by M. Silverstein and G. Urban, 253–276. Chicago: University of Chicago Press.

Merleau-Ponty, Maurice. (1958) 2008. "Rapport de Maurice Merleau-Ponty pour la création d'une chaire d'Anthropologie sociale." In *La lettre du Collège de France,* Hors-série 2. http://lettre-cdf.revues.org/229.

Mestre, Claire. 2006. "La Psychiatrie Transculturelle: Un Champ Necessaire et Complexe." In *Manuel de psychiatrie transculturelle: Travail clinique, travail social,* edited by Marie Rose Moro, Quitterie De La Noë, and Yoram Mouchenik. Paris: La pensée sauvage.

Metzl, Jonathan M., and Helena Hansen. 2014. "Structural Competency: Theorizing a New Medical Engagement with Stigma and Inequality." In *Social Science and Medicine* 103: 126–133.

———. 2018. "Structural Competency and Psychiatry." In *JAMA Psychiatry* 75 (2): 115–116.

Meurs, Dominique, Ariane Pailhé, and Patrick Simon. 2006. "The Persistence of Intergenerational Inequalities linked to Immigration: Labour Market Outcomes for Immigrants and Their Descendants in France." *Population-E* 61 (5–6): 645–682.

Mezzich, Juan, Giovanni Caracci, Horacio Fabrega Jr., and Laurence J. Kirmayer. 2009. "Cultural Formulation Guidelines." *Transcultural Psychiatry* 46 (3): 383–405.

Ministère de la jeunesse et des sports. 2010. "L'histoire des associations." http://www.associations.gouv.fr/article.php3?id_article=1.

Ministère de l'éducation nationale et de la jeunesse. 2012. "Enseignements primaire et secondaire." Bulletin official 37. http://www.education.gouv.fr/pid25535/bulletin_officiel.html?cid_bo=61536.

Ministère de l'intérieur. 2005. "Déplacement de M. Nicolas Sarkozy a Perpignan, 10/13/2005." https://www.interieur.gouv.fr/Archives/Archives-ministre-de-l-Interieur/Archives-de-Nicolas-Sarkozy-2005-2007/Interventions/13.10.2005-Deplacement-de-M.-Nicolas-Sarkozy-a-Perpignan.

Ministère de la justice. 2017. *Rapport annuel d'activité 2016. Mission mineurs non accompagnés.* http://www.justice.gouv.fr/art_pix/RAA_MMNA_2016.pdf.

Ministère des solidarités et de la santé. 2012. *Plan psychiatrie et santé mentale 2011–2015.* https://solidarites-sante.gouv.fr/prevention-en-sante/sante-mentale-et-psychiatrie/article/plan-psychiatrie-et-sante-mentale-2011-2015.

Monfroy, Brigitte. 2002. "La définition des élèves en difficulté en ZEP: Le discours des enseignants de l'école primaire." *Revue française de pédagogie* 140 (July-August-September): 33–40.

Moro, Marie Rose. 2010. *Nos enfants demain: Pour une société multiculturelle*. Paris, Odile Jacob.

Moro, Marie Rose, Quitterie de La Noë, and Yoram Mouchenick, eds. 2006. *Manuel de psychiatrie transculturelle: Travail clinique, travail social*. Paris: La pensée sauvage.

Moro, Marie Rose, Isidoro Moro Gomez, Tahar Abbal, Ameziane Abdelhak, Taieb Ferradji, Francois Giraud, Felicia Heidenreich, Isam Idris, Kouakou Kouassi, Isabelle Real, and Anne Revah-Levy. 2004. *Avicenne l'andalouse: Devenir thérapeute en situation transculturelle*. Paris: La pensée sauvage.

Musée de l'Assistance Publique—Hôpitaux de Paris. 2005. 1935–2005. L'hôpital Avicenne: une histoire sans frontières. Dossier pédagogique. http://www.histoire-immigration.fr/1935-2005-l-hopital-avicenne-une-histoire-sans-frontieres-1.

Myers, Neely Laurenzo. 2015. *Recovery's Edge: An Ethnography of Mental Health Care and Moral Agency*. Nashville: Vanderbilt University Press.

Nail, Thomas. 2015. *The Figure of the Migrant*. Stanford, CA: Stanford University Press.

Nathan, Tobie. 1986. *La folie des autres: Traité d'ethnopsychiatrie clinique*. Paris: Dunod.

———. 1994. *L'influence qui guérit*. Paris: Odile Jacob.

Ndiaye, Pap. 2008. *La condition noire: Essai sur une minorité française*. Paris: Calmann-Lévy.

Nicollet, Albert. 1992. *Femmes d'Afrique noire en France: La vie partagée*. Paris: Harmattan.

Noiriel, Gérard. 1988. *Le creuset français: Histoire de l'immigration au XIXe- XXe siècle*. Paris: Editions du Seuil.

———. 2001. "Les jeunes 'd'origine immigrée' n'existent pas." In *Etat, nation et immigration: Vers une histoire du pouvoir*, 221–229. Paris: Belin.

OFPRA. 2018. *Rapport d'activité*. https://ofpra.gouv.fr/sites/default/files/atoms/files/rapport_dactivite_2018.pdf.pdf

Ong, Aihwa. 1995. "Making the biopolitical subject: Cambodian immigrants, refugee medicine and cultural citizenship in California." *Social Science & Medicine*, 40 (9): 1243–1257.

Ortner, Sherry. 1984. "Theory in Anthropology since the Sixties." *Comparative Studies in Society and History* 26 (1): 126–166.

Pan Ké Shon, Jean-Louis, and Claire Scodellaro. 2015. "L'habitat des immigrés et des descendants: Ségrégation et discriminations perçues." In *Trajectoires et origines: Enquête sur la diversité des populations en France*, edited by Cris Beauchemin, Christelle Hamel, and Patrick Simon, 471–497. Paris: Ined.

Paugam, Serge. 1991. *La disqualification sociale. Essai sur la nouvelle pauvreté*. Paris: Presses Universitaires de France.

Payet, Jean-Paul. 1995. *Collèges de banlieue: Ethnographie d'un monde scolaire*. Paris: Meridiens-Klincksieck.

Péchu, Cécile. 1999. "Black African Immigrants in France and Claims for Housing." *Journal of Ethnic and Migration Studies* 25 (4): 727–744.

Petitjean, F., and D. Leguay. 2002. "Sectorisation psychiatrique: évolution et perspectives." *Annales médicopsychologiques* 160 (10): 786–793.

Policar, Alain. 1997. "La dérive de l'ethnopsychiatrie." *Libération*, June 20, 1997.

Porot, Antoine. 1918. "Notes de psychiatrie musulmane." *Annales médico-psychologiques* 76: 377–384.

Porot, Antoine, and Angelo Hesnard. 1918. *L'Expertise mentale militaire*. Paris: Masson.

Présidence de la République. 2008. "Discours de M. le Président de la République. Une nouvelle politique pour les banlieues." https://www.banquedesterritoires.fr/sites/default/files/ra/Discours%20du%20président%20de%20la%20République%20%3A%20%22Une%20nouvelle%20politique%20pour%20les%20banlieues%22%2C%208%20février%202008.%20.pdf.

Quesada, James, Laurie K. Hart, and Philippe Bourgois. 2011. "Structural Vulnerability and Health: Latino Migrant Laborers in the United States." *Medical Anthropology* 30 (4): 339–362.

Quiminal, Catherine, and Mahamet Timera. 2002. "1974–2002, Les Mutations de l'Immigration Ouest-Africaine." In "Africains, citoyens d'ici et de là-bas." *Hommes et migrations* 1239: 19–32.

Radjack, Rahmeth, Gabriela Guzman, and Marie Rose Moro. 2014. "Enfants mineurs isolés." *Adolescence* 32 (3): 531–539. https://doi.org/10.3917/ado.089.0531.

Réa, Andrea. 2000. *La société en miettes: Epreuves et enjeux de l'exclusion.* Paris: Labor.

Réa, Andrea, and Maryse Tripier. 2008. *Sociologie de l'immigration.* Paris: La Découverte.

Rechtman, Richard. 1995. "De l'ethnopsychiatrie à l'a-psychiatrie culturelle." *Migrations santé* 86: 113–129.

———. 2012. "La psychiatrie à l'épreuve de l'altérité: Perspectives historiques et enjeux actuels." In *Les nouvelles frontières de la société française,* edited by Didier Fassin, 101–127. Paris: La Découverte.

Rezkallah, Nadia, and Alain Epelboin. 2000. *Chroniques du saturnisme infantile 1989–1994: Enquête ethnologique auprès de familles parisiennes originaires du Sénégal et du Mali.* Paris: L'Harmattan.

Ricardou, Rafael, and Samba Yatera. 2007. "Actions collectives et jeunesse(s) 'issue(s) des migrations' subsahariennes en France: Pratiques et expériences du GRDR." *Empan* 3 (67): 112–116.

Robiliard, Denys. 2013. "Des populations oubliées." In *Rapport d'information en conclusion des travaux de la mission sur la santé mentale et l'avenir de la psychiatrie,* 33–34. http://www.assemblee-nationale.fr/14/rap-info/i1662.asp#P707_70791.

Rockwell, Elsie. 2012. "Appropriating Written French: Literacy Practices in a Parisian Elementary School." *Reading Research Quarterly* 47 (4): 382–403.

Rosenberg, Clifford. 2004. "Colonial Politics of Healthcare Provision in Interwar Paris." *French Historical Studies* 27 (3): 637–668.

———. 2006. *Policing Paris: The Origins of Modern Immigration Control between the Wars.* Ithaca, NY: Cornell University Press.

Rostirolla, Daria, and Rachel Wadoux. 2017. "Accueillir la diversité dans le cadre du soin en santé mentale: l'expérience du Centre Minkowska." In *Le défi interculturel. Enjeux et perspectives pour entreprendre,* edited by Pierre Robert Cloet, Alain Max Guénette, Evalde Mutabazi, and Philippe Pierre. Paris: L'Harmattan.

Rouchon, Jeanne-Flore, Reyre Aymeric, Taïeb Olivier, and Marie Rose Moro. 2009. "L'utilisation de la notion de contre-transfert culturel en clinique." *L'Autre* 1 (10): 80–89.

Santiago-Irizarry, Vilma. 2001. *Medicalizing Ethnicity: The Construction of Latino Identity in Psychiatric Settings.* Ithaca, NY: Cornell University Press.

Sargent, Carolyn. 2005. "Counseling Contraception for Malian Migrants in Paris: Global, State, and Personal Politics." *Human Organization* 64 (2): 147–156.

Sargent, Carolyn, and Stéphanie Larchanché. 2009. "The Construction of 'Cultural Difference' and Its Therapeutic Significance in Immigrant Mental Health Services in France." *Culture, Medicine, and Psychiatry* 33: 2–20.

Sargent, Carolyn, and Stéphanie Larchanché-Kim. 2006. "Liminal Lives: Immigration Status, Gender, and the Construction of Identities Among Malian Migrants in Paris." In "Immigrant Identities and the State," edited by Caroline Brettell. Special issue, *American Behavioral Scientist* 50 (1): 9–26.

Sarrandon-Eck, Aline, and Cyril Farnarier. 2014. "Les points rouges ou les critères de l'urgence dans une équipe mobile psychiatrie-précarité." In *La médecine du tri: Histoire, éthique, anthropologie,* edited by Guillaume Lachenal, Céline Lefève, and Vinh-Kim Nguyen, 161–178. Paris: Presses Universitaires de France.

Sauvegrain, Priscille. 2012. "La santé maternelle des 'Africaines' en Île-de-France: Racisation des patientes et trajectoires de soins." *Revue européenne des migrations internationales* 28 (2): 81–100. https://www.cairn.info/revue-europeenne-des-migrations-internationales-2012-2 -page-81.htm.

Sayad, Abdelmalek. 1999. "'Costs' and 'Benefits' of Immigration." In *The Weight of the World: Social Suffering in Contemporary Society*, edited by Pierre Bourdieu et al., translated by Priscilla Parkhurst Ferguson et al., 219–221. Stanford, CA: Stanford University Press.

———. 2004. *The Suffering of the Immigrant.* Cambridge: Polity Press.

Scheper-Hughes, Nancy. 1990. "Three Propositions for a Critically Applied Medical Anthropology." *Social Science & Medicine* 30 (2): 189–97.

———. 1993. *Death without Weeping: The Violence of Everyday Life in Brazil.* Berkeley: University of California Press.

Schiff, Claire. 2012. "En marge du métier, dispositifs d'intégration et pratiques enseignantes face aux élèves primo-migrants en collège." In *Du point de vue de l'ethnicité, pratiques françaises*, edited by Chantal Crenn and Laurence Kotobi, 111–124. Paris: Armand Colin.

Shweder, Richard A. 1991. *Thinking through Cultures: Expeditions in Cultural Psychology.* Cambridge, MA: Harvard University Press.

———. 2003. *Why Do Men Barbecue? Recipes for Cultural Psychology.* Cambridge, MA: Harvard University Press.

Shweder, Richard A., and Robert Levine, eds. 1984. *Culture Theory: Essays on Mind, Self, and Emotion.* New York: Cambridge University Press.

Sibony, Daniel. 1997. "Tous les malades de l'exil." *Libération*, January 30.

Silberman, Roxane, Richard Alba, and Irène Fournier. 2007. "Segmented Assimilation in France? Discrimination in the Labour Market against the Second Generation." *Ethnic and Racial Studies* 30 (1): 1–27.

Simon, Patrick. 2000. "Les jeunes de l'immigration se cachent pour vieillir: Représentations sociales et catégories de l'action publique." *VEI Enjeux* 121: 23–38.

———. 2000b. "Statistics, French Social Science and Ethnic and Racial Relations." *Revue Française de Sociologie* 51: 159–174.

———. 2003. "Le logement social en France et la gestion des 'populations à risques.'" In "France-USA: Agir contre la discrimination." *Hommes et migrations* 1246: 76–91.

Singer, Merrill, and Hans Baer. 1995. *Critical Medical Anthropology.* Amityville, NY: Baywood.

Stengers, Isabelle, and Tobie Nathan. 1995. *Médecins et sorciers: Manifeste pour une psychopathologie scientifique le médecin et le charlatan.* Paris: Les Empêcheurs de penser en rond.

Sturm, Gésine, Thierry Baubet, and Marie Rose Moro. 2010. "Culture, Trauma, and Subjectivity: The French Ethnopsychoanalysis Approach." *Traumatology* 16 (4): 27–38.

Taguieff, Pierre-André. (1987) 2001. *The Force of Prejudice: On Racism and Its Doubles*, translated and edited by Hassan Melehy. Minneapolis, MN: University of Minnesota Press.

Taylor, Charles. 1994. "The Politics of Recognition." *Multiculturalism: Examining the Politics of Recognition*, edited by Amy Gutmann. Princeton, NJ: Princeton University Press.

Terrio, Susan J. 2009. *Judging Mohammed. Juvenile Delinquency, Immigration, and Exclusion at the Paris Palace of Justice.* Stanford, CA: Stanford University Press.

Ticktin, Miriam. 2011. *Casualties of Care: Immigration and the Politics of Humanitarianism in France.* Berkeley: University of California Press.

Tosquelles, F. 2001. "Frantz Fanon et la psychothérapie institutionnelle." *Sud/Nord* 14 (1): 167–174. https://doi.org/10.3917/sn.014.0167.

Tshimanga, Charles, Didier Gondola, and Peter J. Bloom, eds. 2009. *Frenchness and the African Diaspora: Identity and Uprising in Contemporary France.* Bloomington: Indiana University Press.

van Zanten, Agnès. 2009. "Une discrimination banalisée? L'évitement de la mixité sociale et raciale dans les établissements scolaires." In *De la question sociale à la question raciale? Représenter la société française*, edited by Didier Fassin and Éric Fassin, 195–210. Paris: La Découverte.

———. 2012. *L'école de la périphérie: Scolarité et ségrégation en banlieue*. Paris: Presses Universitaires de France.

Vaughan, Megan. 2007. Introduction to *Psychiatry and Empire*, edited by Sloan Mahone and Megan Vaughan, 1–16. New York: Palgrave Macmillan.

Viet, Vincent. 1998. *La France immigrée: Construction d'une politique, 1914–1997*. Paris: Fayard.

Waitzkin, Howard. 1983. *The Second Sickness : Contradictions of Capitalist Healthcare*. New York : Free Press.

Watters, Charles. 2001. "Emerging Paradigms in the Mental Health Care of Refugees." *Social Science and Medicine* 52 (11): 1709–1718.

Weil, Patrick. 2008. *Liberté, égalité, discriminations: L' "identité nationale" au regard de l'histoire*. Paris: Grasset.

Wieviorka, Michel. 2002. *Race, Culture, and Society: The French Experience with Muslims*. In *Muslim Europe or Euro-Islam: Politics, Culture, and Citizenship in the Age of Globalization*, edited by Nezar AlSayyad and Manuel Castells. Lanham, MD: Lexington Books.

Wilkinson, Iain, and Arthur Kleinman. 2016. *A Passion for Society: How We Think about Human Suffering*. Oakland: University of California Press.

Willen, Sarah. 2012. "How Is Health-Related 'Deservingness' Reckoned? Perspectives from Unauthorized Im/migrants in Tel Aviv." *Social Science and Medicine* 74 (6): 812–821.

Willen, Sarah S., and Elizabeth Carpenter-Song. 2013. "Cultural Competence in Action: 'Lifting the Hood' on Four Case Studies in Medical Education." *Culture, Medicine and Psychiatry* 37: 241.

World Health Organization (WHO). 2001. *Mental Health: Results of a Global Advocacy Campaign, World Health Day*. Geneva: World Health Organization.

———. 2010. *mhGAP Intervention Guide for Mental, Neurological and Substance-Use Disorders in Non-specialized Health Settings: Mental Health Gap Action Programme (mhGAP)*. Geneva: World Health Organization.

Young, Alan. 1995. *The Harmony of Illusions: Inventing Post-Traumatic Stress Disorder*. Princeton, NJ: Princeton University Press.

Youssef, Hanafy A., and Salah A. Fadl. 1996. "Frantz Fanon and Political Psychiatry." *History of Psychiatry* 7 (28): 525–532.

Zeroug-Vial, Halima, Yvan Couriol, and Nicolas Chambon. 2014. "Les défaillances de l'accompagnement des demandeurs d'asile et leurs conséquences sur la santé mentale." *Rhizome: Bulletin National Santé et Précarité* 51: 57–60.

INDEX

ABOUT THE AUTHOR

STÉPHANIE LARCHANCHÉ is a medical anthropologist and psychotherapist. She is the director of Research, Teaching, and Professional Training at Centre Minkowska in Paris. She is also a lecturer at Université Paris Descartes and Sigmund Freud University–Paris.

Printed in the United States
By Bookmasters